Improving the Quality
of Care in Nursing Homes

Improving the Quality of Care in Nursing Homes

An Evidence-Based Approach

Thomas T. H. Wan, Ph.D., M.H.S.

Gerald-Mark Breen, Ph.D.

Ning Jackie Zhang, M.D., Ph.D., M.P.H.

Lynn Unruh, Ph.D., R.N.

The Johns Hopkins University Press

Baltimore

The Johns Hopkins University Press
2715 North Charles Street
Baltimore, Maryland 21218-4363
www.press.jhu.edu

Library of Congress Cataloging-in-Publication Data

Improving the quality of care in nursing homes : an evidence-based approach / Thomas T. H. Wan . . . [et al.].
    p. ; cm.
  Includes bibliographical references and index.
  ISBN-13: 978-0-8018-9718-4 (hardcover : alk. paper)
  ISBN-10: 0-8018-9718-1 (hardcover : alk. paper)
  1. Nursing home care—United States—Quality control.
I. Wan, Thomas T. H.
  [DNLM: 1. Quality Assurance, Health Care—methods—United
States. 2. Evidence-Based Medicine—United States. 3. Homes for
the Aged—organization & administration—United States.
4. Nursing Homes—organization & administration—United
States. WX 153 I346 2010]
  RA997.I47 2010
  362.16—dc22   2010001215

A catalog record for this book is available from the British Library.

*Special discounts are available for bulk purchases of this book. For
more information, please contact Special Sales at 410-516-6936 or
specialsales@press.jhu.edu.*

The Johns Hopkins University Press uses environmentally
friendly book materials, including recycled text paper that is
composed of at least 30 percent post-consumer waste, whenever
possible. All of our book papers are acid-free, and our jackets and
covers are printed on paper with recycled content.

Contents

Foreword, by Bernard A. Roos   vii

Acknowledgments   xi

Introduction   Nursing Homes in the United States   1

Chapter 1.   The Quality of Care in Nursing Homes   6

Chapter 2.   Measuring the Quality of Care   17

Chapter 3.   Factors Contributing to the Variability in the Quality of Care   33

Chapter 4.   Persistent Citations for the Deficiency of Pressure Ulcers   46

Chapter 5.   Factors Influencing Residents' Outcomes   59

Chapter 6.   Policies regarding Minimum Staffing Levels   76

Chapter 7.   The Relationship between Efficiency and the Quality of Care   81

Chapter 8.   Improving Performance and the Quality of Life through Health Informatics   90

Conclusion   Synthesis, Prospects, and Future Directions   105

Appendix: Helpful Websites for Clinical Knowledge Management and the Quality of Care   115

References   119

Index   133

Foreword

This volume is a landmark contribution to informing professionals and advocates working for effective, efficient care of nursing home residents.

Professor Thomas T. H. Wan and his coauthors focus on the quality of nursing home care and the disconcerting observation by Grabowski and Castle (2004) that quality remains consistent or does not change significantly in such facilities over time. That is, today's poor- (or high-) quality facilities are also likely to be tomorrow's poor- (or high-) quality facilities. Toward ending this inertia, the authors review past and current views and analyses of the many quality-related factors as well as different aspects and models of nursing home quality and efficiency. The authors progress to a thoughtful perspective on these many factors and issues. Through the lens of their most recent work, the reader can finally envision an exciting solution to quality and efficiency challenges. That solution consists of a universal, systematic introduction and application of information technology and computational science to enhance decision making in nursing homes.

To understand the potential of modeling and informatics to enhance quality and efficiency in nursing homes, this book first reviews evidence related to epidemiologic, social, economic, and financial aspects of long-term care regulation, compliance, and reporting. In discussing this evidence, the authors address the use and helpfulness of consumer complaints for evaluating and ensuring quality. What is unique about this early section is the attention given to understanding the interplay between facility, contextual, and regional influences on quality and efficiency.

Explanation of the major national long-term care datasets (patient-level data from the Minimum Data Set, or MDS, and nursing home quality data from the Online Survey, Certification, and Reporting, or OSCAR, are primary datasets for gauging quality) is followed by a review of their benefits and limitations, as well as some insight into their potential value when used together. The top deficiencies and quality concerns are reviewed, including how they are affected by key performance factors and how they interrelate. This appraisal provides a substantive basis for understanding the need for and potential benefit of providing clinical decision support to enhance staff performance and resident status.

In each chapter, the authors move from background and existing models to identifying specific complexities, introducing new important questions, and proposing innovative approaches to the quality and efficiency of care in nursing homes in the United States. Working toward an analytical model for addressing such complexities and improving performance in our nursing homes, the authors first explicate in detail the resident outcome components of nursing home quality. The components for each key category, such as dignity or physical functioning, are defined and referenced to a specific national dataset (MDS or OSCAR). This initial framework provides an opportunity for multilevel structural equation analysis of the quality of care and opens the way to improved modeling and analysis of quality variations among nursing homes and to understanding how contextual and structural changes affect various outcomes. This framework could be expanded from nursing to include medical, rehabilitation, and social work professional care, leading to a more complete picture of nursing home care and quality. Finally, the authors address multilevel modeling, taking into consideration variation of nursing home quality not only among nursing homes (mainly organizational characteristics) but also among states, which reflects market changes, state regulations, and Medicaid financing.

In working toward the modeling of quality, the authors review contextual, organizational, nurse staffing, and nursing care process in relation to quality-of-care measures and resident states or outcomes. This ambitious attempt succeeds across a wide array of reader backgrounds and training because of a careful stepwise progression of the chapters, beginning with central issues of quality and efficiency and their definition and proceeding to in-depth analysis of their determinants. Chapter 3 is noteworthy for its handling of the relationship between quality and efficiency, not only in general terms but also in the context of care challenges seen in the nursing home. Chapter 7 provides a specific demonstration of the interplay between quality and efficiency and how the existing dataset can afford insights into the potential and opportunities for improving both efficiency and quality.

Chapter 8 lays out the critical and unique prospects for information and education technology to improve quality in nursing homes. The analytic modeling of quality proposed by the authors is feasible within the existing data-collection processes, can be easily validated, and could, for little cost, be applied on a statewide and nationwide basis. The authors emphasize that quality modeling can not only identify the need for specific knowledge, skills, or attitudes, but also trigger the delivery of education and clinical decision support from online clinical education and decision support repositories.

This volume offers hope and is a must-read for anyone interested in the future of institutional care. While information and device technology have entered other care arenas and effectively improved care, this transformation has not yet happened in nursing homes. The authors demonstrate that the fundamental data-collection process capabilities are in place, that their models based on these data are amenable to assessing potential and paths to quality and efficiency improvement, and that the quality and degree of communication can be enhanced by technology. The problem of moving forward with their quality-efficiency improvement strategy has been the lack of positive performance and outcomes expectations related to these factors. This volume goes a long way to creating those positive expectations and to improving the performance of nursing homes nationally.

Bernard A. Roos, M.D.
Professor of Medicine and Director
University of Miami Geriatrics Institute and Miami VA GRECC
Chief Academic Officer, Miami Jewish Home and Hospital
Founder and Director, Florida's Teaching Nursing Home Program

Acknowledgments

This volume and much of the research material within have been partially supported by the National Institute of Nursing Research, National Institutes of Health—research grant R01 NR008226-01A1. We express our earnest appreciation for this significant support in an important, wide-scale project on the quality of care in nursing homes.

Chapter 5 is based on an article previously published by Sage Publications:

> Wan, T. T. H., Zhang, N. J., and Unruh, L. 2006. Predictors of resident outcome improvement in nursing homes. *Western Journal of Nursing Research* 28(8), 974–93.

We appreciate reprint privileges for tables and figures from the following organizations and publishing companies:

The United States Department of Labor

The United States Census Bureau

The Henry Kaiser Family Foundation

Springer Press, for material from the following articles:

> Unruh, L., and Wan, T. T. H. 2004. A systems framework for evaluating nursing care quality in nursing homes. *Journal of Medical Systems* 28(2), 197–214.

> Wan, T. T. H. 2006. Healthcare informatics research: From data to evidence-based practice. *Journal of Medical Systems* 30(1), 3–7.

Health Research and Education Trust, for material from the following article:

> Zhang, N. J., Unruh, L., and Wan, T. T. H. 2008. Has the Medicare prospective payment system led to increased nursing home efficiency? *Health Services Research* 43(3), 1043–61.

The Gerontological Society of America, for material from the following article:

> Bolin, J. N., Phillips, C. D., and Hawes, C. 2006. Differences between newly admitted nursing home residents in rural and nonrural areas in a national sample. *The Gerontologist* 46(1), 33–41.

Anthony J. Jannetti, Inc., for material from the following article:

> Zhang, N. J., Unruh, L., Liu, R., and Wan, T. T. H. 2006. Minimum nurse staffing ratios for nursing homes. *Nursing Economics* 24(2), 78–85.

We are especially grateful for the exceptional editorial work done by Dorothy Silvers. We would like to express appreciation to Wendy Harris, at the Johns Hopkins University Press, for her superb editorial suggestions and to Stan Wakefield for his guidance in selecting an outstanding publisher for us.

Nursing Homes in the United States

Evidence-based research is fundamental to improving the quality of care in nursing homes. Management of the size and capacity of nursing homes, their budgets for resources and for administering care, consistent development of strategies to improve care, and the tools for improving care in general—all these aspects can benefit from the application of evidence-based research on nursing home care.

Since the watershed Nursing Home Reform Act of 1987, which established a federal policy to reduce negligence, abuse of residents, and poor care in nursing homes, little improvement has been documented in nursing home facilities in the United States. Even with the introduction in 2002 of a national Internet-based report card system rating nursing homes, as well as useful databases—Online Survey, Certification, and Reporting (OSCAR) and Minimum Data Set (MDS)—devised by the Centers for Medicare and Medicaid Services (CMS; see www.cms.gov), the quality of life and outcomes for residents are still not being adequately measured or improved. The reliability and validity of these databases and Internet resources have not been addressed satisfactorily. The federal policy effort is also critically undermined by a lack of "teeth" in legislation and its implementation. Nevertheless, valid insights and informed training on how to use available tools, as well as better grounding for those tools, would advance the effort to improve nursing home care.

Upon entering a nursing home, a person's life is so transformed that he or she can be assumed to be in a crisis. The likelihood in the next decades of increasing numbers of elderly persons who have chronic, severe illnesses and functional deficiencies has sharpened attention to the need for nursing research to support the best geriatric health care practices (Breen and Zhang, 2008). That is particularly the case for nursing homes and other long-term care settings, where the need is exigent to improve the quality of care (Newcomer et al., 2001; Maas, Kelley, Park, and Specht, 2002; Scott-Cawiezell et al., 2007).

According to Wang (2007), approximately 2 million Americans reside in 18,000 nursing home facilities and by 2020, another 2 million Americans are predicted to be admitted to one. Currently, 1 percent of those aged 65 to 74, 4 percent of those aged 75 to 84, and 20 percent of those aged 85 or older require almost immediate admission to a nursing home, and they are likely to remain there permanently. The U.S. Department of Health and Human Services (HHS), as cited by Wang (2007), calculated that a person aged 65 or older now has a 40 percent probability of entering a nursing home. Wang states that nearly 5 percent of the elderly population (age $\geq$ 65) enters some kind of nursing home care each year. Making a simple comparative analysis of the nursing home admission rates of women and men over the age of 65, Breen and Zhang (2008) estimate that women are at 45 percent; men are at 28 percent.

Nursing homes in the United States are often viewed as one giant corporation with an extraordinary amount of government involvement (Grabowski and Castle, 2004). The government is the principal purchaser of nursing home care through the Medicaid and Medicare programs. State Medicaid programs account for approximately 50 percent of all nursing home expenditures, and Medicaid recipients use about 70 percent of all bed days. The government also regulates nursing home care, with regulations that apply to nursing homes that accept Medicaid and Medicare recipients (Grabowski and Castle, 2004) and through its surveys and certification. To accept Medicaid and Medicare recipients, a skilled nursing care facility must have an annual certification (stamp of approval) granted after a survey by the CMS. Certified homes must also fill out quarterly MDS assessments for every resident (Mor, 2003; Grabowski and Castle, 2004). Thus, the government acquires an immense amount of information on quality of care at a substantial cost. A recent estimate showed that the survey and certification process costs the government nearly $400 million annually, or about $22,000 per nursing home or $208 per nursing home bed (Walshe, 2001). And that does not include the facility's indirect costs for certification, such as interacting with the regulatory agency, preparing for and hosting survey visits, gathering and providing data, and responding to investigations of complaints. Experience from other sectors of the economy suggests that the nursing home's indirect costs for certification may be higher than the direct costs to the government (Walshe, 2001).

In figure I.1, a Bureau of Labor Statistics (2000) pie chart reveals the fairly

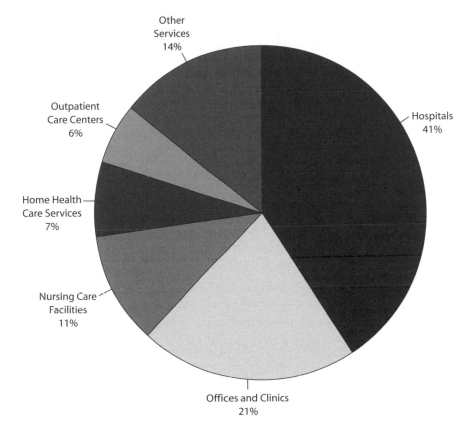

Figure I.1. Employment in the Health Sector, 2000. *Source*: U.S. Department of Labor (2008)

significant portion of employment in health care that is devoted to nursing home care or similar care for elderly or disabled populations. The chart demonstrates the considerable role of nursing home systems and care delivery in U.S. health care.

In 2005, routine annual costs for individualized care in a skilled nursing facility averaged more than $70,000. Annual spending on nursing home care has more than doubled since 1990, to an estimated total of $115 billion in 2004 (Bassett, 2007). Medicare, which covers brief or transient nursing home stays for rehabilitation from acute injury or illness, has seen its share of nursing home costs rise from about 5 percent in 1990 to 16 percent in 2004. Interestingly, Medicare, being restricted to the scope just described, does not cover costs

Table I.1 Ownership and Chain Membership among Skilled Nursing Homes
in the United States, 1997–2003

	Frequency	Percentage
Ownership		
For-profit	42,756	73.05
Nonprofit	13,738	23.47
Government	2,035	3.48
Chain member		
Yes	35,822	61.20
No	22,707	38.80

Source: Zhang, Unruh, and Wan (2008)

for long-term care (Bassett, 2007). Moreover, the share of nursing home costs covered by private insurance and other third-party payers declined from about 15 percent in the late 1990s to about 11 percent in 2004. Partly as a result of the lack of insurance coverage, individuals currently fork out more than 25 percent of their nursing home expenses directly from their private incomes and personal assets. When those who must have nursing home care have exhausted their incomes and assets to pay, they turn to Medicaid (Grabowski, Angelelli, and Mor, 2004). Thus, according to Bassett (2007), Medicaid now covers about 45 percent of annual nursing home costs—an enormous proportion.

Cost-effective care has become crucial for nursing homes throughout the industrialized world (Weech-Maldonado, Shea, and Mor, 2006). Nursing homes face constrained budgets, yet are challenged to provide high-quality care (Scott-Cawiezell et al., 2007). According to Zhang and Wan (2007), the average Medicaid reimbursement rates were $95 and $103 before adjusting for income; 63 percent of nursing homes in 1997 were for-profit, as compared to 62 percent in 2001; 45 percent of the nursing homes in 1997 were chain affiliated; in 2001, 44 percent were chain affiliated.

Zhang, Unruh, and Wan (2008), in an article in *Health Services Research*, presented a table (table I.1) of descriptive statistics on a panel of 8,361 skilled nursing homes for seven years (1997–2003). This panel yielded a total of 58,529 observations for the nursing home care facilities in the United States, including those both licensed and not licensed by CMS, according to ownership and chain membership.

A resident care problem is defined by a deficiency citation for a specific problem observed in a nursing facility's patient care (Wan, 2003). Assessments were made of the outcomes (Wan, 2003) listed next:

1. Freedom from physical restraints
2. Promotion of dignity and respect
3. Accommodation of individual needs and preferences
4. Maintenance of ADL (activity of daily living)
5. Treatment of pressure ulcers
6. Freedom from urinary catheters
7. Treatment of bladder incontinence
8. Freedom from nasogastric tubes
9. Maintenance of acceptable nutritional status
10. Maintenance of proper hydration and health
11. Freedom from unnecessary medications
12. Freedom from significant medication errors

The CMS created a report card system that examines four features of nursing homes' care delivery and patient incidents: (1) worsening abilities to perform daily living skills, (2) new infections, (3) occurrence of pressure ulcers, and (4) number of residents who were physically restrained (Kelly, Liebig, and Edwards, 2008; Castle, 2009).

Any of several sanctions may be placed on facilities that are cited for a high number of deficiencies (a *deficiency* is a term defined in detail in chapter 3). These sanctions may include one or more of the following: (1) civil penalties of up to $10,000 per day, (2) refusal or denial of payment for new admissions, (3) intrusive state monitoring, (4) temporary external and/or increased management, and (5) an immediate injunction terminating operation.

This chapter has described basic features and some key historical aspects of nursing homes in the United States, as well as major issues regarding their current operations. The number of nursing home residents in the United States and the demand for nursing home care, coupled with the competing costs and the federal legislation intended to secure and maintain their ethical integrity, present serious problems. Both collaborative investigation and evidence-based research are needed to bring effective remedies to this volatile area of health care. The next chapter assesses the quality of care in nursing homes in the United States and discusses implications.

CHAPTER 1

The Quality of Care in Nursing Homes

Definitions

Over the past two generations, vast and dispersed increases in the elderly population of the United States have been paralleled by remarkable growth in the nursing home sector as a whole (Forbes-Thompson and Gessert, 2006). Concerns about the quality of care delivered by nursing homes have resulted in an extensive and elaborate system of nursing home regulation and oversight (Putnam et al., 2007), leading some nursing home administrators to refer to nursing homes as "the second most regulated industry in America after nuclear power." In recent years, the quality of life for nursing home residents—which usually does not correspond to or have any congruence with quality of care—has also become a prominent consideration in debates on nursing home policy (Forbes-Thompson and Gessert, 2006; Putnam et al., 2007; Scott-Cawiezell et al., 2007).

According to Grabowski and Castle (2004), the quality of nursing home care (in each facility) is typically consistent, that is, it changes little over time. Today's poor- or high-quality facilities are likely to be tomorrow's poor- or high-quality facilities. This is a disconcerting finding. Regional location, metropolitan size, and the percentage of elderly individuals (75 years of age or older) in the population are pertinent contextual variables for explaining the variation in quality of nursing homes.

According to the Centers for Medicare and Medicaid Services (CMS), nursing home quality is multidimensional, comprising clinical, functional, psychosocial, and other facets of residents' health and well-being (Zhang and Wan, 2005). Historically, however, many studies have used only one or a few indicators of the quality of nursing home care (e.g., mortality rate, resident satisfaction, pressure ulcers). Those limited measures could not adequately reflect the total configuration or "picture" of the quality of care. An alternative way to evaluate the quality of care in nursing homes is to establish a stable and reliable measurement model for evaluating deficiencies. The U.S. Department of Health and Human Services (HHS) defines a nursing home deficiency as a finding that a nursing home failed to satisfy one or more federal or state requirements for care. The number of federal citations for deficiencies in nursing care, made annually by surveyors, is a measure of a home's adequacy.

As the demand for nursing home care increases, so does public pressure to improve quality (Zhang and Wan, 2005, 2007). In a perfect world, registered nurses (RNs) would provide all aspects of care for frail and vulnerable residents; however, in facilities that are struggling with constraints, using staff with a range of credential levels helps guarantee care that is cost effective as well as of adequate quality (Roy and Mor, 2005; Scott-Cawiezell et al., 2007). Setting out to monitor and strengthen the quality of care in nursing homes, researchers over the past 20 years have developed and adjusted the definition and measurement of quality. At first, simple quantitative measures of quality prevailed, such as staff hours per resident day (Elwell, 1984) or changes in residents' physical functioning (Linn, Gurel, and Linn, 1977; Newcomer et al., 2001). Moos and Lemke, in the early 1980s, developed a Multi-Phasic Environmental Assessment Procedure (MEAP), a multidimensional assessment that factors in characteristics of the residents and staff, physical features of the facility, policies, and social climate (Zhang and Wan, 2005, 2007).

One must recognize, however, that a resident's evaluation of the quality of care is subjective. Every resident in a particular nursing home may receive the same quality of care, yet each may perceive differences in its quality. In individual nursing homes, perhaps asking each resident to evaluate the quality of care from his or her perspective, and then combining all the responses in that facility, may enable an interpretation of the overall quality of care there. R. A. Kane and R. L. Kane (1988), for example, proposed a multidimensional approach to assess the outcomes for residents: amalgamating self-reported data with the data from investigator interviews. Six health concepts or dimensions were assessed: (1) cognitive, (2) affective, (3) social activities, (4) activities of daily living, (5) resident satisfaction, and (6) physical functioning.

Stevenson (2006) presented the first national research using consumer complaints to evaluate—and to ensure—the quality of care in nursing homes. Despite limitations, complaints about nursing homes record real-time signals of lapses in the quality of care, albeit from the resident's viewpoint. Consumer complaints correspond strongly with objective quality measures and point to the trajectory of nursing home quality between survey visits. Records of complaints are an additional, low-cost method for policy makers to monitor the quality of care in nursing homes, and they give the public salient information for also doing so. As processes for investigating complaints and for data monitoring draw increased interest and examination, the trustworthy complaints in terms of both assessing and ensuring the quality of care should rise. Perhaps that will help improve the quality of care and the quality of life for nursing home residents (Putnam et al., 2007; Goodson, Jang, and Rantz, 2008).

General Information

For several decades, the quality of care in nursing homes has raised concern (Unruh and Wan, 2004; Putnam et al., 2007) due to reports of inadequate, negligent, or abusive care and the associated litigation. Hence, nursing homes have come under increasing scrutiny and regulation. Their quality of care has been of great concern to both the public and the private sectors (Mullan and Harrington, 2001; Putnam et al., 2007; Scott-Cawiezell et al., 2007). Since 1959, a Senate subcommittee, a Department of Health, Education and Welfare investigation, several state studies, three Institute of Medicine studies, a series of legal actions, five Health Care Financing Administration (HCFA)–financed demonstration projects, and numerous other researcher-initiated projects have produced a flood of information about the reform of resident care (Wan, 2003; Mor, 2005). Thus, for years, an array of committees and agencies has investigated a range of aspects of the quality of nursing home care and has instigated governmental oversight and regulation (Institute of Medicine, 1986, 1996, 2001; U.S. Department of Health and Human Services, 1999; Putnam et al., 2007).

Between 1990 and 1999, the quality of care in nursing facilities did improve somewhat, though not adequately. The average number of deficiencies per facility in the United States dropped from 7.9 in 1991 to 5.4 in 1999 (Walshe and Harrington, 2002). Unsatisfactory quality of care, failure to provide comprehensive care plans for residents, and poor resident assessment remained among the top ten deficiencies cited by state surveyors in the twenty-first century (Harrington et al., 2000a, 2000b; Putnam et al., 2007).

Data from the Minimum Data Set (MDS), a resident-based assessment tool (Mor, 2003), and the Online Survey Certification and Reporting (OSCAR) systems have been used in nursing home research (Wan, 2003; Bellow and Halpin,

2008). OSCAR is a national database of nursing homes in the United States that includes critical specifics (Mullan and Harrington, 2001; Zhang, Unruh, Liu, and Wan, 2006; Scott-Cawiezell et al., 2007). OSCAR information covers three areas: (1) characteristics of the facility, including all categories of nurse staffing; (2) resident census and health conditions; and (3) deficiency measurements (Zhang, Unruh, Liu, and Wan, 2006). All nursing home facilities federally certified for Medicare and Medicaid are included in this data system, except for those in the trust territories and Puerto Rico. State inspectors collect OSCAR data every 9 to 15 months to verify nursing homes' compliance with all federal and state regulations. It should be borne in mind that nursing homes self-report on the second category, resident health conditions. In table 1.1, Unruh and Wan (2004) provide an example of the use of OSCAR data to delineate the contextual and structural components of the quality of care in nursing homes.

The Center for Health Systems Research and Analysis (CHSRA) of the University of Wisconsin, and the Nursing Home Case Mix and Quality Demonstration (NHCMQ), have developed 37 quality indicators (QI) from the MDS in 12 care domains, which have been tested and found to be good indicators of nursing home quality of care (Rantz et al., 1997; Putnam et al., 2007). In general, both researchers and clinicians recommend the use of MDS to measure improvement in the quality of nursing homes' care (Mor, 2003; Phillips, Chen, and Sherman, 2008).

Published studies that have used OSCAR or similar data include Harrington et al. (2000a, 2000b), Mullan and Harrington (2001), and Hendrix and Foreman (2001). Those studies assessed resident outcomes: pressure ulcers, incontinence, resident behavior, quality of life, observance of residents' rights, and mortality. Other commonly used measures are process indicators such as use of restraints, skin care, catheterizations, and ombudsperson programs.

OSCAR data are considered accurate reflections of actual deficiencies (Harrington et al., 2000a, 2000b). Several approaches have been taken to apply OSCAR deficiency data. Harrington et al. (2000a, 2000b) group deficiencies into three broad categories: (1) quality of care, (2) quality of life, and (3) other. This process has the advantage of reducing variability due to the surveying process. Mullan and Harrington (2001) classify OSCAR data into eight highly correlated domains or factors of deficiencies. Their analyses use a single wave of data; however, validation of the quality of care construct that uses deficiencies as negative indicators of quality should employ multiwave data. Specifically, longitudinal analysis of indicators of nursing care quality should determine the

Table 1.1 Components of the Quality of Care in Nursing Homes

Component	Available data
Contextual components	
Population characteristics (% aged; % female; % white)	Area Resource File
Population health status	
Per capita or median income of the county	
Location: urban vs. rural, region and state	
Market competition (County Herfindahl Index)	
Supply of nursing homes	
Regulatory constraints (CON, BBA)	
Medicaid, Medicare, private reimbursement type and rate	
Organizational factors/facility characteristics	National nursing
Bed size	surveys; OSCAR
Ownership	
Chain affiliation	
Number of Medicaid days	
Payment mix	
Case mix	
Certification status	
Average ADLs of residents	
Percent skilled nursing residents in a nursing home	
Nurse staffing, education, and proficiency	OSCAR
Registered nurses (RNs) per 100 residents	
Licensed practical nurses (LPNs) per 100 residents	
RN–nurses ratio	
Nursing hours per 100 residents	
Nurse assistant (NA) training	
RN, LPN, NA proficiency	
Nursing administration	

Source: From "A systems framework for evaluating nursing care quality in nursing homes" Table 1 of Unruh and Wan (2004, p. 202). With kind permission of Springer Science and Business Media.
  Note: ADL = activity of daily living; BBA = Balanced Budget Act; CON = certificate-of-need; OSCAR = Online Survey, Certification, and Reporting system.

stability of the measurement instrument (Wan, 2003). Further, the effect of nursing care processes on the quality of care should be examined in multiple waves of OSCAR data.

Zhang and Wan (2005) confirm from a number of earlier empirical and government publications (Institute of Medicine, 1986; Zimmerman et al., 1995; Harrington, 2001b) that the nation has an unacceptably high percentage of nursing homes with low-quality care. Breen and Zhang (2008) concur with that assertion and supporting measured observations.

Several health and gerontology scholars have reported that nonprofit facilities deliver better quality of care than for-profit ones do (Unruh, Zhang, and Wan, 2006; Zhang and Wan, 2007; Breen and Zhang, 2008). Chain membership of nursing homes has been associated with lower quality of care in some studies (e.g., Harrington et al., 2000a). Whether the facility is hospital-based has been taken into consideration in several studies, but these results have been inconsistent. The negative impact of certain facility characteristics, in particular the percentage of residents receiving Medicaid, has been shown to have a major bearing on the quality of care. Policy makers debating future cuts in Medicaid or Medicare spending for nursing home care should consider such features of the resident population (Unruh, Zhang, and Wan, 2006).

The organizational factors of bed size, ownership, chain affiliation, payment mix, and average acuity level of residents are considered to influence the quality of care in nursing homes. Other research has found that for-profit facilities have fewer professional nurses and a lower quality of care, and receive more federal deficiency citations than nonprofit facilities do. Because approximately 67 percent of U.S. nursing homes are for-profit, that finding is alarming. Finally, resident acuity is important to consider in the analysis, because rising acuity levels of residents require more extensive and intensive interventions (Wan, Zhang, and Unruh, 2006; Zhang and Wan, 2007).

Staff Interpersonal Communication Skills

In high-risk health care environments, the basic interpersonal skill to communicate with a special population is indispensable for the relationships between medical practitioners and patients (Barry, Brannon, and Mor, 2005; Intrator et al., 2005; Arnold and Boggs, 2006; Breen and Matusitz, 2008; Matusitz and Breen, 2007; Breen and Zhang, 2008; Breen et al., 2009). Otherwise, the quality of care, as measured by resident satisfaction as well as by outcomes and deficiencies in care delivery are all likely to be affected negatively, whether directly or indirectly. Particularly in nursing homes, having basic social and psychological needs met sufficiently to ensure resident satisfaction as well as improve outcomes should be a top priority (Breen and Zhang, 2008). In particular, improving the quality of "life" of elderly nursing home residents by reducing depersonalization requires attention to their individual losses and suffering. The staff working in nursing homes directly caring for diverse and complex human beings must be capable of understanding how residents' suffering is rooted in their lifelong experiences and personal perceptions, and of demonstrating that awareness. Individualized admission assessments ought to transcend the medical diagnoses, skin assessment, and pharmacy review, to incorporate assessments of feelings of loss and grief, the potential for depression, and recognition of residents' individual coping strategies (Forbes-Thompson and Gessert, 2006; Scott-Cawiezell et al., 2007).

Staff on the forefront of care delivery can be guided to appreciate the roles they have in preventing or ameliorating suffering, with particular attention to steps that contribute to maintaining the dignity, individuality, and personhood of residents (Forbes-Thompson and Gessert, 2006). Such training can occur during basic education for their respective roles and also in continuing education. Certified nursing assistants (CNAs), in particular, should be trained to place the common and urgent demands of residents into the context of residents' loss and their attempts to maintain human dignity, rather than viewing their demands as a burden (resident) to be avoided.

That sort of attention to individualized, resident-focused assessment and care and relevant staff training are being addressed in some nursing homes by the rapidly growing, grassroots movement referred to as "culture change" (Forbes-Thompson and Gessert, 2006). Nursing homes undertaking culture change espouse daily attention to resident choice; empowerment of workers on the forefront, who know the resident best; creative care techniques; fostering human relationships by using regular staff assignments; reducing boredom through a broader variety of activities; fostering meaning and purpose through the care of pets; making milieus more homelike by structural changes to living arrangements; and facilitating the organizational and functioning of team work in nursing homes. These ideas and changes are being widely embraced, but there exists little evaluative information on how and to what extent adopting these changes makes a significant difference in meeting the psychosocial needs and improving the quality of life of residents (Forbes-Thompson and Gessert, 2006; Scott-Cawiezell et al., 2007; Temkin-Greener et al., 2009).

Ethnicity and the Quality of Care

In 2004, the work of Grabowski (2004) and of Cashen, Dykes, and Gerber (2004) revealed certain overwhelming facts about race and ethnicity, and nursing home care in the United States. Their work was followed by other important articles supporting their revelations (Mor et al., 2004; Angelelli, Grabowski, and

Table 1.2 The Nursing Home Population, by Age Group, Race/Ethnicity
(in percentages)

Race/Ethnicity	Age Group			
	55–64	65–74	75–84	85+
American Indian and Alaskan Native	51.7%	30.0%	14.6%	3.6%
Asian and Pacific Islander	51.1	30.0	16.1	2.9
Black	46.7	33.0	16.1	4.3
Hispanic	50.6	30.6	14.7	4.1
White	42.1	30.1	21.6	6.2

Source: From "A systems framework for evaluating nursing care quality in nursing homes" Table 3 of Unruh and Wan (2004, p. 204). With kind permission of Springer Science and Business Media

Mor, 2006; Miller et al., 2006; Breen and Zhang, 2008). This research has revealed that African Americans are disproportionately admitted to low-quality nursing homes that have high numbers and high frequencies of deficiencies. In a standard comparison of Caucasian and African American populations admitted to nursing home facilities, Grabowski (2004) discovered that, after controlling for resident and home characteristics, African Americans entered nursing homes that had 44 percent more deficiencies (mean = 7.39) than found in nursing homes with mostly Caucasian admissions (mean = 5.13).The study also found conclusive evidence that Hispanics were admitted to nursing home facilities that had 43 percent more deficiencies (mean = 7.33) than nursing homes caring mostly for Caucasians. Further, of the remaining residents—who represented "other" ethnicities—the results indicated that they were admitted to nursing homes that had 35 percent more deficiencies (mean = 6.94) than the average found for all admissions.

Table 1.2 provides a fairly recent account of the percentages of residents in nursing homes according to ethnic group. The age ranges also show notable trends related to ethnicities in the percentages of people from each age group across the lifespan that enter nursing homes.

Long-term care (LTC) is a critical, ongoing problem for many American Indian tribes. The Indian Health Service (IHS), the primary source of health care for rural American Indians, provides minimal LTC, leaving the tribes themselves struggling to finance and provide more adequate services themselves (Jervis and Manson, 2007). In fact, only a small fraction of the 561 federally recognized tribes own and operate nursing homes. Undertreatment for psychiatric disorders is thought to be more prominent and serious for nursing home residents who are ethnic/racial minorities than for the general population (Mor et al., 2004; Angelelli, Grabowski, and Mor, 2006; Miller et al., 2006). That may be particularly the case for American Indian residents. Given the barriers to mental health care erected by poverty, rurality, and dependence on the under-funded IHS, American Indian residents are often undertreated for such conditions (Jervis and Manson, 2007).

Rural Nursing Homes

Rural nursing home populations tend to be older and poorer, and to have less insurance coverage (Coward, Duncan, and Netzer, 1993). In addition, rural nursing homes usually are smaller, have fewer hospital-based facilities, have a smaller proportion of Medicare recipients, and tend to have more difficulty re-cruiting and retaining nurses. Rural nursing home residents typically are older (median = 88) and Caucasian. Generally they have higher percentages of do-not-resuscitate orders and living wills, and their nursing home stays are usually covered by Medicaid. Rural nursing home residents are also more likely to have been hospitalized at some point before their final three months of life (Gessert et al., 2006).

Earlier research findings about rural nursing homes suggest that individ-uals admitted to rural nursing homes generally have lower care requirements and that rural facilities are differentiated by their combinations of short-term and long-term residents (Bolin, Phillips, and Hawes, 2006). Also, rural nursing homes are sometimes more likely to receive residents who are cognitively im-paired (Mitchell et al., 2003; Wu et al., 2005a). Because these residents have greater tendencies toward behavioral problems, nursing staff members who are trained to manage these special problems are in high demand. Among residents who are not receiving Medicare, noticeably more have significant cognitive impairment in rural nursing homes. There are fewer frail residents, however, meaning residents with decreased acuity levels. Rural nursing home residents also are less likely to die in the hospital than are their urban counterparts (Levy, Fish, and Kramer, 2004). Interestingly, Coburn, Bolda, and Keith (2003) find higher rates of nursing home use among rural residents than among residents in other geographically defined locations.

A study by Bolin, Phillips, and Hawes (2006) demonstrated a variety of major differences between residents admitted to urban and those admitted to rural nursing homes. First, a higher proportion of those entering rural facilities are

Table 1.3 Individuals Admitted to Nursing Homes, by Location of the Nursing Home

Type of Admission	Location of the Nursing Home				
	Urban	Large Town	Small Town	Isolated	Total
All admissions (n; %)	149,003; 75	23,116; 12	17,283; 9	8,187; 4	197,589; 100
Medicare admissions	104,913; 70	17,661; 76	11,693; 68	4,768; 58	139,035; 70
Non-Medicare admissions	44,090; 30	5,455; 24	5,590; 32	3,419; 42	58,554; 30
Total (%)	100	100	100	100	197,589

Source: Bolin, Phillips, and Hawes (2006)

non-Medicare admissions: for the nation as a whole, Medicare recipients constitute 70 percent of all admissions, but in small towns and isolated areas, they constitute less than 65 percent of admissions. The results also show that new nursing home residents in rural areas are older, more likely to be White, and less likely to enter a nursing home from an acute-care setting. This research, on a national sample of newly admitted nursing home residents, supports the general conclusion that rural facilities have residents with acuity scores lower than for those in urban nursing homes (Bolin, Phillips, and Hawes, 2006).

Table 1.3 shows data on the variation in types of coverage in nursing home locations across the United States. The table also shows the percentages of nursing homes located in rural areas.

Persons admitted to rural or isolated nursing homes are more likely to be clinically stable and have a lower likelihood of death, and to have less activity of daily living (ADL) impairment than do those admitted to urban facilities (Jervis and Manson, 2007). However, rural facilities are somewhat more likely to have an admission of a cognitively impaired individual, who has potential behavior problems, than are urban facilities (Mitchell et al., 2003; Bolin, Phillips, and Hawes, 2006). This particular problem may be exacerbated in rural nursing homes, because of a lack of mental health specialists and because rural residents' presentation of depressive symptomatology may differ from the usual (Jervis and Manson, 2007).

Previous research offers various hints about the factors that might generate the study results described above (Bolin, Phillips, and Hawes, 2006; Zhang and Wan, 2007). Rogers (1997) found that rural elderly people are more likely than other elderly people to be living alone by the age of 75, which is when the likelihood of a nursing home admission increases. Rural elderly individuals are also more likely than urban elderly individuals to be poor, and thus unable to pay for help that might extend their time at home (Coburn and Bolda, 1999; Bolin, Phillips, and Hawes, 2006). Some research also reveals that nursing home residents in rural areas report more frequently than their urban counterparts do that needed services were not accessible to them in their communities or were optional (Coward, Duncan, and Freudenberger, 1994; Bolin, Phillips, and Hawes, 2006).

In an environment of profit-seeking and bottom-line business mentalities, rural nursing homes represent only mildly interesting markets for those managed care companies that have ample resources to extend overall institutional capacity and perhaps improve the quality of care. In many rural nursing home markets, there may be limited options for care (Newcomer et al., 2001; Grabowski and Castle, 2004). Because there are generally fewer medical providers as well as insufficient number of residents to constitute a lucrative venture for external entrepreneurs, rural nursing homes appear unappealing to managed care companies (National Association of Rural Health Clinics, 1998). Managed care organizations find it hard to negotiate discounts with rural nursing homes, rendering any plans for cooperation between them less financially secure and competitive.

This chapter has provided a general introduction to issues in the quality of care in U.S. nursing homes. There are resources available to examine the quality of the care delivered in nursing homes, such as the OSCAR and MDS databases. The chapter also has discussed the interpersonal communication skills that nursing home staffs have and should improve. The differences in the quality of care in nursing homes according to the predominant racial and ethnic groups they admit have been discussed.

CHAPTER 2

Measuring the Quality of Care

Given the change in reimbursement mechanisms occurring as the baby-boomers age, the quality of the care in nursing homes has become even more of an urgent concern. Since 2000, a score of empirical, scholarly studies and government reports have documented the low quality of care found in nursing homes (Grabowski, 2001; Harrington, 2001a, 2001b; Wan, 2002; Wan and Connell, 2003; Unruh and Wan, 2004; Zhang and Wan, 2005, 2007). Working with medically frail residents of nursing homes is challenging: their medical problems are often unstable, and mood and activity level can fluctuate unpredictably with pain and infection (Newcomer et al., 2001; Wu et al., 2005b; Meeks et al., 2006). One example of the challenges involved—the intense nature of early morning care with the multiple activities of washing, dressing, grooming, continence care, and transfer assistance—is depicted by Sloane et al. (2007). The authors suggest that the relatively short time allotted to that care (9 to 15 minutes, depending on the facility) implies that care providers must rush; residents have little chance to rest, relax, or relish the personal attention in one-on-one care. Finally, a major component of the difficulties residents and their caregivers face is the fact that most residents have suffered many serious losses not only in health, and perhaps cognition, but also in their personal relationships, independence, and finances (Forbes-Thompson and Gessert, 2006).

The literature suggests a series of reasons for the dismal record of nursing home care. Some studies have emphasized that state constraints, especially the level of Medicaid reimbursement, are associated with the low quality of care in nursing homes (Grabowski, 2001; Bassett, 2007; Putnam et al., 2007). Other researchers and policy makers have pointed their fingers at the lack of reliable and validated measurement as one hurdle to improving quality of care in nursing homes (Harris and Clauser, 2002).

Most previous studies have evaluated the effects of federal and state regulations on nursing homes at the facility level. Though valuable, facility-level analysis alone is not adequate to assess the overall consequences of regulation (Zhang and Wan, 2005, 2007). Because nursing homes within one state are affected by the same policies, the within-state variation of nursing home quality cannot be explained by the differences in regulations, such as Medicaid reimbursement and certificate-of-need (CON). As a matter of fact, the state should be the unit of analysis for evaluating state regulations. Hence, nursing home quality should be measured at the state as well as the facility level (Zhang and Wan, 2005).

The serious concerns and the recent availability of national databases on nursing home deficiencies have inspired extensive study of the state-level measurement model of nursing home quality (Scott-Cawiezell et al., 2007). Without specifications of the causal factors influencing nursing home care, it is impossible to form effective strategies for improving quality of care. Better understanding of the relationships of key contextual and facility factors with the quality of nursing and rehabilitative care is needed (Wan, Zhang, and Unruh, 2006; Zhang and Wan, 2007).

An external environmental factor may influence not only nursing home performance but also the quality of care, through its influence on structural variables. According to Unruh, Zhang, and Wan (2006), the 1997 Balanced Budget Act (BBA), mandating a Medicare prospective payment system (PPS) for skilled nursing facilities, has had negative consequences for their licensed nurse staffing and their quality of care.

The Medicare PPS for skilled nursing facilities (SNF) was implemented to reduce nursing home costs by aligning reimbursement with resource use intensity. The initial payment system was phased in over four years starting in 1998, with the fixed prospective portion increased by 25 percent each year (Zhang, Unruh, and Wan, 2008). The effects were greater on staffing than on quality, which suggests that the worsening of care was due partly to reductions in staffing. If so, simply increasing the reimbursement for staffing might not solve that problem, because many other factors influence staffing and also the quality of care (Konetzka, Stearns, and Park, 2008).

In 1999, the Balanced Budget Reconciliation Act, and in 2000, the Benefits Improvement and Protection Act attempted to mitigate the financial strain on facilities from the 1997 BBA. The new legislation, which increased baseline payments in 2000 and 2001, respectively, had positive effects on both the staffing levels and resident outcomes in nursing homes (Wan, Zhang, and Unruh, 2006; Zhang, Unruh, and Wan, 2008). Notably, the percentage of residents receiving Medicaid was shown to affect both staffing and quality negatively (Unruh, Zhang, and Wan, 2006). However, another study (Bassett, 2007) on the effect of the 1999 Medicaid reimbursement rate did not show any impact on staffing and the quality of care. Although the proportion of Medicaid in the payer mix independently influences the quality of care negatively, when combined with the BBA's reductions in Medicare reimbursement, it tempers their impact, probably because facilities with higher proportions of Medicare recipients are more affected by the Medicare reimbursement cuts (Unruh, Zhang, and Wan, 2006). Other factors also can influence staffing levels and the quality of care (Konetzka, Stearns, and Park, 2008). For example, the shortage of nurses could affect staffing levels, independently of the changes in reimbursement system (Zhang and Wan, 2007).

Instruments for Measuring the Quality of Care

Wan measured the quality of nursing care using multiple indicators of nursing home structure, process, and resident outcomes as well as state agencies' yearly assessments of nursing home deficiencies (Wan, 2003). A one-factor or unidimensional measurement model for each of two quality constructs was verified by the data in each study year. This empirical study of the relationship between adequate staffing levels of nursing care and the quality of the care demonstrated that a positive relationship exists between the process and outcome dimensions of the quality of nursing care (Wan, Zhang, and Unruh, 2006). The quality of care in nursing homes can be benchmarked at the facility and state levels by using the underlying measurement model. The results of facility deficiency comparisons can then guide selection of a nursing home (Zhang and Wan, 2005). The federal government can refer to the results of state-deficiency comparisons to adjust policies for resource allocation and Medicaid reimbursement.

In another approach, studies frequently cited in the literature on quality measurement use instruments designed and developed by expert panels (Zhang and Wan, 2005). Twenty-seven patient-related problems were specified in a study on the processes of care (Shaughnessy et al., 1995; Zhang and Wan, 2005). The Quality Assessment Index (QAI) developed by Gustafson et al. (1990) came up with seven components of the quality of care. Most of the early studies on patient care were individual efforts. Since the Omnibus Budget Reconciliation Act in 1987, however, federal involvement has established national data and facilitated more reliable methods. The U.S. Department of Health and Human Services (HHS) developed a comprehensive patient assessment instrument, the MDS, to collect uniform patient information on all nursing home residents who receive patient care planning (Zhang and Wan, 2005, 2007). The MDS uses more than 400 items to measure a range of clinical, functional, behavioral, and social attributes of nursing home residents. All Medicare- and Medicaid-certified nursing facilities are required to report MDS items for their residents at least every three months. The Centers for Medicare and Medicaid Services (CMS) gathers data for all states. Originally designed as a care-planning tool, MDS is now applied in research and used to generate or identify quality indicators (Zhang and Wan, 2005; Scott-Cawiezell et al., 2007).

Since the early 1990s, the Health Care Financing Administration (HCFA) has contracted with the Center for Health Systems Research and Analysis (CHSRA) at the University of Wisconsin to establish and test a set of MDS-based indicators of nursing home quality indicators (QIs) of care (Philips, Hawes, and Fries, 1993). The Wisconsin study built on Zimmerman's Quality Assessment Index (ZQAI). Eventually, 24 QIs were developed, for four domains of care: functional, clinical, psychosocial, and pharmacological. CHSRA has completed validation studies for these QIs that found they had high accuracy ratings (Zhang and Wan, 2005, 2007).

OSCAR (Online Survey, Certification, and Reporting) is the principal national source for data on nursing home quality (Zhang and Wan, 2005). As a surveillance system, it has been used to evaluate compliance by nursing homes with federal and state regulations. The General Accounting Office [(GAO) 1999] and Mullan and Harrington (2001) reported that OSCAR data are generally validated and reliable. However, systematical validation of these data has yet to be empirically executed. State inspectors apply both process and outcome measurements to assess the quality of care in nursing homes. The process measures evaluate whether appropriate procedures are used in nursing home care as regulated by the CMS (Zhang and Wan, 2005). The outcome measures examine negative outcomes such as pressure ulcers. A deficiency citation is given to a facility when it fails to meet a standard. Obviously, more deficiencies represent lower quality (Breen and Zhang, 2008). OSCAR is explained in detail in the next section.

Online Survey, Certification, and Reporting (OSCAR)

Much deficiency data for each nursing home is drawn from the OSCAR database system. All U.S. facilities federally certified for Medicare and Medicaid are included in the OSCAR database, except for those located in the trust territories and Puerto Rico. State inspectors collect OSCAR data every 9 to 15 months to verify compliance with all federal and state regulations. OSCAR has 185 deficiency items in 17 categories (Zhang and Wan, 2005).

OSCAR contains four areas of information: facility characteristics, resident census, conditions of residents, and deficiency measurements. The 17 major categories of quality measurements used in surveys are:

1. Resident rights
2. Admission, transfer, and discharge rights
3. Resident behavior and facility practices
4. Quality of life
5. Resident assessment
6. Quality of nursing and medical care
7. Nursing services
8. Dietary services
9. Physician services
10. Rehabilitation services;
11. Dental services;
12. Pharmacy services;
13. Infection control;
14. Physical environment;
15. Administration;
16. Laboratory services
17. Others

In addition to measurements of quality, OSCAR includes other useful information: on nursing home structure (e.g., bed size, staffing, hospital affiliation, services offered) (Konetzka, Stearns, and Park, 2008); on resident case mix (e.g., proportion of residents requiring assistance with activities of daily living or who are incontinent); on payer mix (Medicare, Medicaid, or others); on system membership (multifacility affiliation and name); on quality assurance (QA) management (QA committee and approved training program); as well as on many health and non-health-related deficiencies reported by state inspectors (Zhang and Wan, 2005).

The accuracy, validity, and reliability of the OSCAR data have been previously examined and reported by government agencies and researchers. A GAO (1999) report found that the OSCAR data were generally reliable. The OSCAR data have become a widely applied tool in research on long-term care. They have been used for improving quality (Unruh and Wan, 2004), evaluating the association between nurse staffing and quality (Harrington et al., 2000a, 2000b; Konetzka, Stearns, and Park, 2008), assessing nursing home quality of care under the restraints of Medicare and Medicaid policies (Zinn et al., 2003; Bassett, 2007), and establishing strategic interventions to improve nursing home quality of care (Castle, 2003a).

Errors have been reported in the survey and rating system of the OSCAR database (Zhang and Wan, 2005). Social, economic, and political factors may influence or skew the survey validity and reliability (Mullan and Harrington, 2001). Therefore, it is generally believed that resident-level data are better for representing the quality of care in nursing homes. With resident-level data such as the MDS available for analysis, the clustering of residents in a facility should be handled in multilevel modeling. In the future, MDS data linked with OSCAR data could gauge the stability of a three-level measurement model of nursing home quality. Indeed, multilevel measurement modeling may become the methodological foundation for evaluating the effectiveness of state regulations and evidence-based practice in nursing homes (Zhang and Wan, 2005, 2007).

The Structure-Process-Outcome Model

The quality of care in nursing homes is multidimensional (Unruh and Wan, 2004), because it must comprise not only clinical (medical and nursing) care, but also social and environmental support of the residents [i.e., their quality of life; Glass (1991), Breen and Zhang, (2008)]. All these aspects of quality are interconnected. For example, good nursing care depends in part on the environment in which the nurses work and the residents live. The interaction of these dimensions of care results in resident outcomes that is likewise multidimensional. Residents need to have their basic needs met, but also need a decent quality of life (i.e., social and emotional health; Breen and Zhang, 2008). Therein lies the complexity of defining the quality of care in nursing homes and of identifying the factors that influence it.

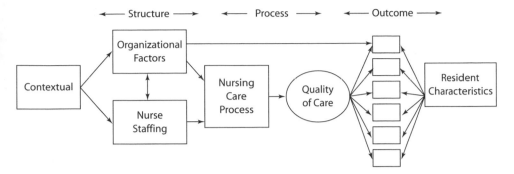

Figure 2.1. The Structure-Process-Outcome Model of the Quality of Care in Nursing Homes. *Source*: From "A systems framework for evaluating nursing care quality in nursing homes" Figure 1 of Unruh and Wan (2004, p. 209). With kind permission of Springer Science and Business Media

Although the quality of care in nursing homes has been studied for decades (Unruh and Wan, 2004), frameworks to guide this line of research are only now emerging. Generally, the models eschew the Donabedian structure-process-outcome (SPO) framework common in research on the quality of care by physicians or hospitals (Cho, 2001; Unruh and Wan, 2004; Zhang and Wan, 2007), or they adjust it so it is better suited to the nursing home environment.

The SPO framework (Donabedian, 1988) is a theoretically informed approach to the longitudinal study of the quality of care. In the Donabedian (1988) framework, structural measures of quality are the professional and organizational resources available to provide care. Process measures are things done to and for patients by health care practitioners. Outcomes are the patient states resulting from the care processes.

Frequently, each of these three components in the Donabedian model is used separately as an indicator of quality. In other studies, the structural factors are causally linked to patient outcomes or processes of care. Rarely is each component perceived as causally related to each other (i.e., structure is related to process, which is related to outcome). Even less commonly does the SPO framework model interrelationships between components (Unruh and Wan, 2004).

Unruh and Wan (2004), in the *Journal of Medical Systems*, presented an SPO systems model of the quality of nursing care in nursing homes. Figure 2.1 demonstrates how the various factors in nursing homes weave together to form this SPO model.

The earliest models for the quality of care in nursing homes appeared in 1991. Glass (1991) believes that the Donabedian framework is inadequate when applied to long-term care. She emphasizes four dimensions of general nursing home quality: (1) staff intervention, (2) physical environment, (3) nutrition/food service, and (4) community relations. For each dimension, two subdimensions are identified; for example, staff intervention has these subdimensions: quality of care and quality of caring (Unruh and Wan, 2004).

Atchley (1991) believes that the Donabedian framework is misapplied in a cross-sectional view. Structure, process, and outcomes transpire not simultaneously, but in a time-ordered process. Atchley has delineated an SPO system in which input factors lead to actions or procedures over time, which then render outcomes over time, and each of these feeds back into the other.

Sainfort, Ramsay, and Monato (1995) discussed the importance of understanding the causal linkages between the structural, process, and outcome factors that produce the quality of care in nursing homes. They urged an understanding of the direct links between the organizational (structural) characteristics under management control and process or outcome indicators. Managerially controllable factors ("organizational slack") comprise staffing, direct care expenditures, case mix, and social services consultants.

Organizational slack factors are important to study because they are the most controllable, are likely to vary from institution to institution, and may differ as a result of influence from other organizational characteristics such as ownership status, size, chain affiliation, or other factors in the operating environment (Unruh and Wan, 2004; Zhang and Wan, 2007). In contrast to how most studies tackle the issue of causality, in this model the organizational slack factors mediate between other organizational factors, and process or outcomes, so the impact of those factors on process or outcomes is indirect.

Rantz et al. (1999b) designed a non-SPO, multidimensional, theoretical model for nursing home quality of care, based on results from focus groups of nursing home staff and residents in Missouri nursing homes. The authors' integrated model identifies these dimensions of quality: adequate and caring staff, positive communication, a safe and pleasant environment, family involvement, a compassionate atmosphere, and a homelike environment. Residents, families, staff, and community are all focal points of these dimensions.

Employing a model originally created by Porras (1987), Stevenson et al. (2000) categorize the overall quality of a nursing home into four interacting dimensions of the organizational environment: (1) organizing arrangements, (2) social factors, (3) technology, and (4) physical setting. These organizational factors are used to identify problems that harm the quality of care in nursing homes, according to the authors' review of nursing home studies using these factors. For each of these four dimensions, the combined influence of these factors on the nursing care process or resident outcomes has not been explicitly examined.

To some degree, Stevenson et al. (2000) discuss interactions between organizational factors. One such example, as described in Unruh and Wan (2004), is that authoritarian managerial styles discourage communication, and poor communication and inadequate training for nursing assistants lead to misunderstandings and dissatisfaction, and consequently, to high turnover. Therefore, although not explicitly elaborated, this model has an affinity with the SPO framework (Zhang and Wan, 2007).

One other framework, by Mueller (2000), focuses narrowly on nurse staffing to assist managers in analyzing nurse staffing needs and their solutions. The author envisions a framework for staffing that begins with the establishment of standards and a philosophy of care, then identifies residents' needs, and from those needs determines the required quality and quantity of nursing personnel, then allocates the nursing personnel and the delivery of care, and ends up with residents' needs being met in accord with the standards and the philosophy of care (Mueller, 2000; Unruh and Wan, 2004; Scott-Cawiezell et al., 2007).

Given the need for a systems framework that explores the causality and complexity of nursing home care, a version of an SPO model could be an improved framework (Unruh and Wan, 2004). However, the existing SPO-like models are somewhat limited, particularly when considered separately. Shortcomings of the models include theses: (1) not linking all three components of the SPO framework; (2) not considering the influence of intra-organizational forces such as leadership and administrative practices on climate and culture; (3) not accounting for the influence of contextual factors, particularly the market, on structural factors; and (4) not accounting for intrastructural linkages (Zinn and Mor, 1998).

Proposed Elements of an Expanded Structure-Process-Outcome (SPO) Framework

In the original SPO framework elaborated by Donabedian (1988), the quality of health care comprises components that pertain to the organizational characteristics of health care providers (structure), the clinical and nonclinical processes involved in care delivery (process), and the effect of care on the health status of patients and populations (outcomes). More precisely, structure refers to the health care setting—the physical facilities, equipment, and other physical resources, and the financial status; also the human resources, including physicians, nurses, dietitians, environmental workers, therapists, and other personnel (Unruh and Wan, 2004; Zhang and Wan, 2007). Structure also includes the organization of the physical and human resources, as well as their quality. For example, in terms of nursing resources, structure is concerned with the nursing care model and the quantity, skills, and education of the nursing staff.

Process pertains to the activities carried out by the health care management and the staff, including their communications and interactions with each other and the patients, and the things they do to or for patients that contribute to the patients' health and well-being. For nursing care in particular, process includes its assessment, planning, delivery, and evaluation (Unruh and Wan, 2004).

Outcomes refers to patient health and welfare—management of pain, patient satisfaction, and functional status, as well as chronic illness, recovery from illness, and mental and social health (Wu et al., 2005b). The outcomes can be either positive states such as relief from pain, improved functional status and freedom from illness, or negative states such as untreated pain, acquired infections, and injuries (Unruh and Wan, 2004).

Factors not considered in the original SPO framework are the external environment's influences on health care providers and institutions (Unruh and Wan, 2004). These are the social, legal, and political contexts in which providers and institutions function, such as government regulations, market competition, and conformity to customs and rules (Fottler, 1987). The external environment exerts influence both through demands placed on the organization and through norms and myths that the organization absorbs. Sociological institutional theory identifies these pressures as coercive, normative, and mimetic (Powell and DiMaggio, 1991). These pressures can be considerable. Consider, for example, the impact of the BBA of 1997 on provider organization (Turnbull, 2000). The act reduced reimbursement to health care providers in nearly every delivery area, making new demands for efficiency ("coercive pressure"). These changes were a continuation of normative changes taking place throughout the 1980s that gave nonproviders more control over delivery decisions ("normative pressure"). Yet, an organization's response to the BBA depended in large part on how other organizations responded: for example, as to whether the organization reduced its staffing ("mimetic pressure"). Because the external environment can thus have a significant impact on the internal one, the SPO framework proposed in this volume includes a precursor category of contextual or institutional components of quality (Unruh and Wan, 2004).

Nor are the influences of residents' characteristics—age, sex, case mix, or acuity considered in the original SPO model. Yet, to properly link context, structure, and process to outcomes (directly or indirectly), any contribution to outcomes by the residents' own status should be considered (Arling et al., 1997). Hence, it is appropriate to include a final set of factors that reflect the residents' characteristics (Unruh and Wan, 2004; Zhang and Wan, 2007).

For nursing facilities, the contextual/institutional components are the socioeconomic and demographic characteristics of the population, the relevant market, the location, reimbursement mechanisms and rates, and regulatory control. Socioeconomic and demographic factors routinely examined in the literature are the median income of the county and population characteristics such as age, sex, and health status (Spector, Selden, and Cohen, 1998). Per capita income is also considered because it suggests the possible percentage of self-paying residents in the area, which could increase the demand for better quality care (Spector, Selden, and Cohen, 1998; Newcomer et al., 2001; Unruh and Wan, 2004).

Metropolitan and state location, differences in case mix, Medicare and Medicaid payment systems (Bassett, 2007), regulations, and oversight practices are other contextual components (Swan et al., 2000). Differences among states with regard to their survey practices also affect the processes of quality assessment and data collection (Unruh and Wan, 2004). Market factors such as the level of competition are explored for their motivation of quality improvement (Castle and Fogel, 1998).

A Structure-Process-Outcome (SPO) Framework for Evaluating the Quality of Care

The linkages outlined above in the empirical literature indicate the paths in a total systems framework for nursing home quality. Although most of the studies described do not connect all the parts of the framework, when their linkages are combined and extended, a more complete and systematic framework can emerge (Unruh and Wan, 2004).

In the expanded SPO framework proposed here, linkages between context and structure, structure and process, and process and outcomes are the main channels among the components. Several of these direct "conduits" from one component to another are also simultaneously indirect paths, traveling through another component first; for instance, the path of context to outcomes goes through structural and process components.

Contextual factors directly influence organizational factors and nurse staffing and indirectly influence other components through a chain of events going all the way to resident outcomes (Zhang and Wan, 2007; Konetzka, Stearns, and Park, 2008). Even though studies indicate direct linkages from context to process and outcomes, it seems probable that these are indirect linkages, as indicated by the model, except for components such as case mix that have a direct effect on resident outcomes (Unruh and Wan, 2004).

The empirical literature shows how important nurse staffing is as a structural factor, and it should be separated from other structural factors, particularly organizational characteristics (Konetzka, Stearns, and Park, 2008). The separation is important because several structural components influence staffing (i.e., intrastructural linkages exist). One example of this is the relationship between ownership and staffing levels (Unruh and Wan, 2004). Moreover, nursing staff levels and competency may feed back into the organizational structure of the facility; for instance, staff adequacy or inadequacy can affect size, payer mix, or costs. The feedback or bidirectional relationships have not been researched. Sainfort, Ramsay, and Monato (1995) list other probable intrastructural linkages, including urban setting and payer mix. These considerations are indicated in the proposed model by placing nurse staffing in a separate box with double arrows going to organizational components.

Organizational factors and nurse staffing directly affect the process of nursing care. Organizational factors such as case mix directly affect resident outcomes (Zhang and Wan, 2007). Other organizational factors, such as facility size and ownership, are not modeled as direct links to resident outcomes even though empirical studies indicate a direct relationship because the linkage is more likely indirect through the influence of organizational factors on nurse staffing and the nursing process (Unruh and Wan, 2004).

Unruh and Wan, in their *Journal of Medical Systems* article (2004), presented a table (table 2.1) that delineates the various components of resident outcome, based on available data from the MDS and OSCAR databases. These indicators are important for evaluating the quality of nursing home care.

Nursing care processes are influenced by several sources, including contextual ones (indirectly) and organizational ones (directly), and these in turn

Table 2.1 Components of Resident Outcome

Resident outcome category	Resident outcome component	Available data
Quality of life	To be free from physical restraints To engage in ongoing activities that fit the resident	MDS[a] OSCAR[b]
Human dignity and self-determination	To be able to choose activities, schedules, interact with members of community, and make choices about aspects of life in the facility	OSCAR
Freedom from abuse	To be free from verbal, sexual, physical and mental abuse, corporal punishment, and involuntary seclusion	OSCAR
Safety/prevention of injury	Prevalence of any injury Prevalence of falls	MDS
Clean environment	To have a safe, clean, comfortable, and homelike environment	OSCAR
Individualized care	To have individual needs and preferences accommodated	OSCAR
Physical functioning	Prevalence of bedfast residents Incidence of contractures	MDS
Urinary/GI tract health	Prevalence of indwelling catheters Prevalence of bladder or bowel incontinence Prevalence of bladder/bowel incontinence without a toileting pan Prevalence of urinary tract infections Prevalence of fecal impaction	MDS
Nasogastric tubes	Prevalence of tube feeding	MDS
Proper nutrition and hydration	To have acceptable nutritional status To have proper hydration Prevalence of weight loss Prevalence of dehydration	OSCAR, MDS
Appropriate medication use	Freedom from unnecessary drugs Freedom from significant medication errors	OSCAR, MDS
Freedom from chemical restraint	Freedom from chemical restraint for purposes of discipline or convenience Prevalence of antipsychotic use in the absence of psychotic and related conditions Prevalence of antipsychotic daily dose > guidelines Prevalence of antianxiety or hypnotic use Prevalence of hypnotic use on a scheduled basis or pro re nata more than two times in the past week Prevalence of antibiotic and anti-infective use Use of 9 or more scheduled medications	

(*continued*)

Table 2.1 *Continued*

Resident outcome category	Resident outcome component	Available data
Cognitive, emotional and behavioral health	Prevalence of problem behavior toward others	OSCAR,
	Prevalence of symptoms of depression	MDS
	Prevalence of symptoms of depression, with no treatment	
	Incidence of cognitive impairment	
Skin status	Prevalence of stage 1 to 4 pressure ulcers	MDS

Source: Unruh and Wan (2004).
[a]Quality indications obtained from the Minimum Data Set (MDS)
[b]Online Survey, Certification, and Reporting System (OSCAR)

influence resident outcomes. The effects of nursing processes on outcomes are one way of viewing the quality of care. Thus, the proposed model delineates a quality of care construct that is a latent component bordering on both process and outcomes. Finally, the model includes resident characteristics, especially those not captured in case mix that influence resident outcomes directly (Newcomer et al., 2001; Unruh and Wan, 2004; Zhang and Wan, 2007).

Missing from this model are other components of nursing home quality of care—the role of medical, ancillary, and assisting personnel in non-nursing processes: medical care and rehabilitation, as well as environmental and social support. These processes also affect resident outcomes. Unruh and Wan's (2004) study did not include physician care or supportive services because the study focused on nursing care. There are few empirical studies of the relationship of the clinical care by physicians to the quality of care in nursing homes.

The type of theoretical SPO framework elaborated above requires an analytical model capable of handling its complexities. A multilevel structural equation analyzing the quality of care in nursing homes would be appropriate for this framework. That would improve the statistical modeling of nursing home quality of care and could reconcile analytical differences in accounting for its variation. Such modeling could be effective for investigating both the direct and the indirect effects of contextual and structural changes on each of the processes and outcomes that delineate the components of the quality of care. In the future, the framework elaborated here should be further expanded to include other aspects of the quality of care in nursing homes, particularly the care provided by physicians in rehabilitation; and environmental and social support as well. Empirical studies that have dealt with those non-nursing aspects of care should be reviewed to extract the contextual, structural, process, and outcome components and their linkages. Inserting them in this framework would reveal a more complete picture of the quality of care and resident quality of life (Unruh and Wan, 2004).

Multilevel Confirmatory Factor Analysis of Panel Data

Zhang and Wan's (2005) study validates the measurement model of nursing home quality by applying multilevel confirmatory factor analysis. The results demonstrate that the two-level measurement model is necessary because nursing homes are clustered at the state level. Their findings lend further support to and bolster the validity of this measurement model of nursing home quality.

Methodological developments, especially the techniques for analyzing hierarchical data, encourage the application of two-level modeling (Zhang and Wan, 2005). As Mullan and Harrington (2001) discussed in their published work, nursing homes are nested within three hierarchies: (1) inspectors, (2) states, and (3) census regions. This pattern suggests the need to perform multilevel analysis to evaluate state variations in nursing home quality of care. Zhang and Wan's (2005) study systematically examines the two-level measurement model. It also establishes a revised state-level measurement model.

The newly established state-level measurement model of nursing home quality of care reduces the measurement from eight categories to seven categories of quality. The low factor loading of "assessment" in the state-level model indicates little variability in assessment deficiencies. That situation suggests homogeneity in the performance of resident assessments. The consequent elimination of the "assessment" indicator has improved the fit of the state-level measurement model to the data.

Two-level factor modeling by Zhang and Wan (2005) represents the variation in the quality of care not only among nursing homes, but also among states. The variation in quality of care among individual nursing homes results more from organizational characteristics; however, given the fact that 75 percent of nursing home care is financed by Medicaid, the variation of nursing home quality of care among states results more from market changes and state regulations (Bassett, 2007). From a theoretical perspective, neither the market nor the regulation differences among states can be disregarded or overlooked. State market differences include the percentage of the elderly population, average household income, and market competition. State regulation includes constraints by CON authorization and reimbursement levels. To study how market and regulation factors affect nursing home quality of care, examination and establishment of a two-level measurement model is extremely important (Zhang and Wan, 2007).

The quality of care in nursing homes can be standardized at the facility and the state levels using the underlying measurement model. As pointed out earlier, comparing facilities' deficiency results can guide the choice of a facility by members of the public. The federal government can use state deficiency comparison results to adjust resource allocation and Medicaid reimbursement policy.

In forthcoming work in this area, MDS data, linked with OSCAR data, could evaluate the stability of a three-level measurement model of nursing home quality. Last, multilevel measurement modeling may become the methodological foundation for evaluating state regulations and evidence-based practice in nursing homes (Zhang and Wan, 2005, 2007).

This chapter has provided detailed information on how researchers, experts, and practitioners measure the quality of care in nursing homes. The instruments most often used have been discussed. OSCAR was identified and explained, as a database of reported quality-of-care ratings in nursing homes in the United States. Expansion of the SPO model was examined for its application to evaluating the quality of care in nursing homes. More details on the dimensions or factors contributing to the variability of care quality in nursing homes are examined in the next chapter.

CHAPTER 3

Factors Contributing to the Variability in the Quality of Care

Citations for Deficiency

Nursing homes are essentially institutional care settings. As businesses, they contend with market forces, facility management issues, and payment and reimbursement problems, as well as with resident characteristics and cultural composition which profoundly influence the quality of care in any nursing home. Health care administration of nursing homes, in general, and quality of care, in particular, can be variously affected according to the diverse dimensions involved.

Nursing home facilities are intended to house, protect, serve, and help rehabilitate people with serious medical ailments (Zhang et al., 2006; Castle and Engberg, 2007b; Breen and Zhang, 2008; Breen et al., 2009). Yet, many nursing home facilities still lack the features needed to perform these functions. Mounting empirical evidence describes the end of life in nursing homes as fraught with problems: pain, unavoidable weight loss, dehydration (Wu et al., 2005), pressure ulcers, and family stress (Forbes-Thompson and Gessert, 2006). To describe such flaws or inadequacies in nursing homes, scholars and gerontologists use the term *deficiency*.

According to the U.S. Department of Health and Human Services (2004, p. 34), a deficiency is "a finding that a nursing home failed to meet one or more federal or state requirements." Common and recurring deficiencies in nursing homes revolve around diminished care, resident dissatisfaction, and less-than-satisfactory resident outcomes. The frequent use of restraint devices (Straker, 1999; Castle, 2002; Breen and Zhang, 2008); catheterizations for urinary or fecal incontinence (Robinson, 2000; Mullan and Harrington, 2001); the development of pressure ulcers (Zhang et al., 2006); the presence of contractures (Clay, 2007); or the improper dispensing of psychoactive medications (Liperoti et al., 2005; Castle and Engberg, 2007b; Vogelsmeier, Scott-Cawiezell, and Zellmer, 2007) are all measures of deficiencies.

According to the Kaiser Family Foundation (2009), ten common and major deficiencies are found in nursing homes in the United States. They are (1) accidents and failures in (2) food sanitation, (3) quality of care, (4) professional standards, (5) accident prevention, (6) housekeeping, (7) comprehensive care plans, (8) infection control, (9) dignity, and (10) pressure sores. Much of what table 3.1 reports about deficiencies overlaps with what other professional researchers have documented.

In terms of quality measures, the incident rates of certain conditions constitute deficiencies. For example, Unruh, Zhang, and Wan (2006) identify incident rates of residents with catheters, physical restraints, and pressure sores. They also consider mortality rate and patient satisfaction as indications of either sufficient or deficient care (Zhang and Wan, 2005, 2007; Unruh, Zhang, and Wan, 2006). The Centers for Medicare and Medicaid Services (CMS) post a comprehensive stipulation of the quality of care as "multidimensional, encompassing clinical, functional, psychosocial, and other aspects of resident health and well being" (Morris et al., 2003).

Improper dispensing of medications is a significant indication of poor nursing home care. Some nursing homes use medications inappropriately, especially mind-altering substances or psychoactive medications (Castle and Engberg, 2007b; Scott-Cawiezell et al., 2007; Vogelsmeier, Scott-Cawiezell, and Zellmer, 2007). Hence, exploring and scrutinizing medication use in nursing homes continues to be important. One research approach is to examine the structural factors and market factors associated with receiving any of these deficiency citations. There is a dearth of data on the probability that a facility receiving a deficiency citation will receive one again in the future. Therefore, a second research approach is to examine the structural and market factors associated with receiving repeated deficiency citations. The safety of medication delivery in nursing homes in the United States is under serious scrutiny as attention to medication errors grows (Barker et al., 2002; Vogelsmeier, Scott-Cawiezell, and Zellmer, 2007). Most nursing home residents have more illnesses and are prescribed more medications than those in community-based care. These residents are subject to higher risks for adverse effects. The consequences of medication errors made in nursing homes can be subtle and evolve

Table 3.1 The Top Ten Deficiencies in U.S. Nursing Homes, 2005

Deficiency	Percentage
Food sanitation	35
Quality of care	29
Professional standards	28
Accidents	23
Accident prevention	22
Housekeeping	22
Comprehensive care plans	20
Infection control	17
Dignity	16
Pressure sores	16

Source: Data from www.statehealthfacts.org/comparemaptable.jsp?ind=419&cat=8

gradually. Such errors frequently have greater consequences than are reported in other long-term care settings (Scott-Cawiezell et al., 2007).

Castle and Engberg's (2007b) study explores two research concerns: deficiency citations about regular medication use and deficiency citations about the use of psychoactive medication. Nursing home residents often are prescribed four times as many medications as noninstitutionalized elders (Walley and Scott, 1995). That makes the possibility of medication errors a legitimate concern (Handler et al., 2006; Vogelsmeier, Scott-Cawiezell, and Zellmer, 2007). A medication error is defined as a dose that is not the same as on the medication order. Interruptions and distractions are often associated with the occurrence of medication errors (Scott-Cawiezell et al., 2007). These authors define distractions as events that do not stop medication administration but as those that divert the medication administrator's attention. Interruptions are events that discontinue the administration of medication.

The prescribing of psychoactive drugs in nursing homes is a particular problem (Lakey et al., 2006). Psychoactive drugs affect emotional function and behavior. Appropriately dispensed in nursing homes, they can reduce acute agitation and emotional distress. Historically, these drugs have been used excessively to control disruptive behavior and nocturnal restlessness and have become known as "chemical restraints" (Unützer and Bruce, 2002). Their efficacy for long-term use has not been established. Moreover, these medications are frequently associated with prescription errors and adverse events (Castle and Engberg, 2007b). The varied levels of credentialing among nursing home staff challenges the safe administration of medications.

The results found by Castle and Engberg (2007b) showed that from 1997 to 2003, on average, 10.8 percent of facilities received psychoactive-specific deficiency citations, 24.7 percent received medication error deficiency citations, and 24.6 percent received medication administration deficiency citations. The correlations between these categories were less than 0.4. The authors also found that in two or more years from 1997 to 2003, 10.1 percent of facilities received psychoactive-specific deficiency citations, 10.6 percent received medication error deficiency citations, and 17.6 percent received medication administration deficiency citations (Castle and Engberg, 2007b). Confidence intervals at 95 percent were found for the multinomial logistic regression models examining the deficiency citations for medication use from 1997 to 2003.

Examining the results for the organizational factors, Castle and Engberg (2007b) concluded that bed size was associated with receiving more deficiency citations across all three groups of citations. For example, with a 10 percent increase in bed size, facilities were 13 percent more prone to receive a psychoactive-specific deficiency citation. The average percentage of Medicaid occupancy also was associated with the probability of receiving more deficiency citations across all three groups of citations. The authors' hypotheses about staffing patterns received mixed support. High levels of RN (registered nurse) staffing were usually associated with less likelihood of receiving deficiency citations, whereas high levels of licensed practice nurse (LPN) or NA (nurse assistant) staffing were not significantly associated.

A market factor, the level of Medicaid reimbursement rates, was associated with the likelihood of fewer deficiency citations across all three groups of citations. For instance, with a $50 increase in the Medicaid reimbursement rate, facilities were 40 percent less likely to receive a psychoactive-specific deficiency citation (Castle and Engberg, 2007b). Castle and Engberg (2007b) also found no support for their hypotheses examining market resources.

The Size of the Staff

An expert panel of the Joint Commission on Accreditation of Healthcare Organizations (JCAHO) reports that nursing shortages pose serious risks to health care, threatening the general quality of care (Joint Commission on Accreditation of Healthcare Organizations, 2002; Scott-Cawiezell et al., 2007). The JCAHO report shows that 90 percent of nursing homes have too few nurses to provide even the most basic of care and shows conclusively the need for a thorough investigation of nurse staffing and how it affects the quality of care in nursing homes (Wan, 2003).

"The positive relationship between nurse staffing levels and the quality of nursing home care has been demonstrated widely" (Zhang et al., 2006, p. 1). Zhang and Grabowski (2004) found support for their theory that the relationship between staffing and quality may be nonlinear. Hendrix and Foreman (2001) also supported that finding. In a nonlinear relationship, minima and maxima may be identifiable. Zhang et al. (2006) examined the minimum nurse staffing thresholds necessary to achieve both quality and efficiency in nursing homes. Zhang et al (2006) and earlier studies corroborate the quality of care in nursing homes demands more financial resource allocation to nurse staffing than often is customary. Registered nurse staffing has been strongly identified as a remedy to deficiencies in nursing home care (Harrington et al., 2000a, 2000b).

One nonlinear framework for defining nursing staffing standards is an economic approach that uses a production function to model the relationship between staffing and quality (Smyth, 1991; Hendrix and Foreman, 2001; Newcomer et al., 2001). Production functions provide information about the optimum level (that is, quantity) of output given increases in one input such as labor. In the usual production function, the relation is nonlinear and S-shaped; the S-shaped relationship reflecting the marginal (that is, incremental) changes in quantity given marginal changes in the labor input: as labor inputs increase, quantity increases first at a faster, then at a slower rate, and at some point stops increasing altogether. In economic theory, the optimum level of production is in the region of decreasing marginal returns to labor. An exact optimum can be determined when the production function is combined with cost data (Zhang et al., 2006; Zhang and Wan, 2007).

From the viewpoints of both improving the quality of care and efficiency, the desired nurse staffing point is hypothesized to be in the area of diminishing marginal returns. From the standpoint of quality improvement, this is the range at which care is still improving. From the standpoint of efficiency, this is the range at which cost efficiency returns to additional staffing are still positive (Zhang et al., 2006). The minimum point of operation is the spot at which the marginal returns shift from increasing to decreasing. The maximum point of operation is the spot at which the returns shift from decreasing marginal to diminishing total returns. The minimum point in this range is the minimum nurse staffing level to maintain both reasonable quality and reasonable efficiency in nursing facilities. By identifying the minimum staffing point in this range, we can establish the staffing point below which both quality and efficiency suffer (Zhang et al., 2006).

To control cost and thus enhance efficiency, nursing homes strive to identify what the plausible minimum staffing levels are to satisfy high quality of care. It has been a challenge to ascertain the best evidence-based minimum staffing ratios and then to institute them. If increasing nurse staffing improves the outcomes of nursing home care, identification of recommended nurse staffing levels becomes crucial as well as achievable (Zhang et al., 2006; Zhang and Wan, 2007).

Zhang et al. (2006) conducted a study that explored the minimum nurse staffing thresholds necessary to achieve both quality and efficiency in nursing homes. The study used a concept of the minimum nurse staffing based on organizational efficiency, which relates nurse staffing as input and nursing home quality as output. This efficiency-oriented notion identifies the staffing threshold above which the growth rate of nursing home quality decreases—the starting point of the decline of a quality return on additional investment in staffing. This efficiency-oriented minimum for nurse staffing is critical because it represents a joint position in which the quality of care and efficiency converge (Scott-Cawiezell et al., 2007). These results, too, are in line with earlier studies that found that better quality of care in nursing homes requires more investment in nurse staffing (Zhang, et al., 2006; Harrington and Swan, 2003).

A study conducted by Zhang et al. (2006), published in *Nursing Economics*, presented a figure (figure 3.1) that depicts the production function of quality of care and nurse staffing (for instance, quality of care and returns with respect to nurse staffing).

Zhang et al. (2006) found indications that the relationship between staffing and quality is not linear, and that a point can be ascertained at which adding additional nursing staff, though it continues to improve quality, does so at a declining rate. That point can be used to establish the minimum staffing necessary to maintain quality of care at 50 percent, 75 percent, and 90 percent levels of quality. The results from the Zhang et al. (2006) study demonstrate that to reach higher levels of quality, minimum staffing requirements surge. The 75 percent quality ranking requires much more nurse staffing for all categories of staff than the 50 percent ranking does. However, moving from 75 percent to 90 percent does not involve as substantial an increase. The reason may be that the quality of care level that would justify an attainable minimum level of staff is

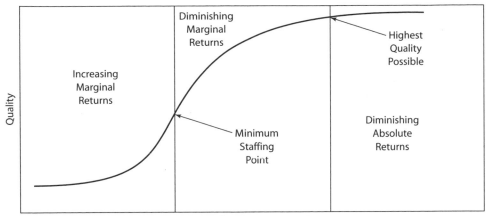

Figure 3.1. The Production Function of Quality of Care and Nurse Staffing. *Source:* From "Minimum nurse staffing ratios for nursing homes" Figure 1 of Zhang et al. (2006, p. 80). With kind permission of Anthony J. Jannetti, Inc.

somewhere between 50 percent and 75 percent. In that case, future studies should assess the minimum staffing requirements for between 50 percent and 75 percent rankings of the quality of care (Zhang et al., 2006).

Research on minimum nurse staffing has two clients: governments and nursing home administrators (Zhang et al., 2006). Federal and state governments use the research as a reference to adjust their surveillance and their reimbursement policy. Nursing home administrators use it as a reference to guide their personnel management and the extent of their quality improvement. The study conducted by Zhang et al. (2006) offers the government minimum nurse staffing values based on fairly current national data. These values should be updated yearly, given changes in policies, quality indicators, and technological advances. Because of regional and facility variations, it would not be appropriate for nursing home administrators to use the minimum nurse staffing values directly. Instead, these values can be used as a national benchmark against which each nursing home could establish its own levels of adequacy.

Residents' Integrity

In the context of nursing home residents, integrity refers to a resident's personal fulfillment and self-respect, individual values and desires, and general togetherness (Kihlgren, Hallgren, and Norberg, 1994; Granerud and Severinsson, 2003; Scott-Cawiezell et al., 2007). Integrity also implies that a resident has control and direction over his or her life and individualized treatment. In cases of extended care, the preservation of integrity is deemed a principal precondition for high quality of care, highlighting an ethical aspect of nursing home care. Preserving the resident's integrity requires dignified treatment by the staff (Robinson, 2000): a clear awareness and appreciation of each resident's history, values, desires, and traditions. Also, because the physical, psychological, social, and spiritual/religious aspects of nursing home residents are salient and interwoven, integrity is of pivotal importance to resident satisfaction and outcomes (Powers, 2005). Teeri et al. (2007), for example, discovered a significant positive correlation between residents expressing their desires to nursing staff and their psychological treatment.

Depression is prevalent in nursing homes and has numerous negative implications for care burden, functional status, cognitive status (Mitchell et al., 2003; Wu et al., 2005a, 2005b), medical morbidity, and mortality (Meeks et al.,2006). Prevalent cognitive and medical comorbid conditions significantly complicate treatment in nursing homes. Further, characteristics of the nursing home environment interact with personal disability and dysphoria (feeling unwell) to create powerful maintaining factors by decreasing personal control and increasing reinforcement for dependency. Individual interventions from outside the nursing home may be temporarily effective, but treatment gains may deteriorate rapidly once external consultation is withdrawn (Meeks et al., 2006). Although research has demonstrated that medical and psychosocial interventions for depression can be effective among elderly people in general, there is a paucity of research demonstrating the effectiveness of interventions for depression in nursing home residents.

An emphasis on increased pleasant activity for nursing home residents is similar to the behavioral activation component of cognitive therapies for depression (Scott-Cawiezell et al., 2007). Empirical support for an activity-related intervention in nursing homes also stems from a body of evidence accumulated by Lawton (1997) that links depression to resident activity level, affective tone of activities, and levels of positive and negative affect.

Residents' families voice opinions of what they have seen in nursing homes concerning resident integrity. Relatives notice that residents are prone to lonesomeness and isolation and that they lack opportunities for leisure activities.

Teeri et al. (2007) assert that resident loneliness is oftentimes a corollary of excessive solitude. Residents who experience seclusion and unmet social needs commonly suffer a personal sense of meaninglessness, which can easily compromise resident social integrity. Hence, more residents' relatives are pressuring staff members to increase opportunities for residents to socialize and find enjoyment (Granerud and Severinsson, 2003).

Researchers have presented evidence that nursing home residents are less likely to experience death, pressure ulcers, dehydration, or urinary tract infections if a family member or friend visits them in the first month of their stay. The fact remains that nursing home residents are predominantly elders with no informal family support to serve as advocates (Grabowski and Castle, 2004).

The Size of the Nursing Home

Although, as noted above, a larger facility size has been associated with a higher rate of deficiencies (Unruh, Zhang, and Wan, 2006), the impact on staffing is less conclusive: some studies find that large facilities have lower levels while others have higher levels. Castle (2002) asserted that smaller nursing homes oftentimes have fewer accessible resources. Yet, smaller nursing homes may be better equipped to tailor to the needs of each resident. Harrington and Swan (2003) contend that there is a familiarity that permeates or exists in smaller nursing homes, whereby social relationships can better form between staff and residents. Hughes, Lapane, and Mor (2000) promote increased relational bonding between staff and residents in smaller nursing homes, and empirically found that small facility size has a positive association with the quality of care. Further, Castle and Engberg (2007b) believe that smaller nursing homes are associated with fewer deficiency citations. Smaller, nonprofit and non-chain-affiliated facilities have fewer lawsuits brought against them (a proxy for poor quality); a higher incident rate of lawsuits is positively associated with deficiency citations (Wan, Zhang, and Unruh, 2006). As a result, it should be declared that promoting and establishing more, smaller nursing homes, that is, homes with sizes that appropriately, adequately, and proportionately meet the needs of every resident—should lead to greater resident integrity, satisfaction, and outcomes. Future research should explore whether better outcomes are consistently associated with smaller facility size.

Residents with Cognitive, Psychological, and/or Motor Dysfunction

Not surprisingly, cognitive, psychiatric, and/or behavioral problems are common in nursing homes (Mitchell et al., 2003; Wu et al., 2005b). They are among the most widespread diagnoses made on nursing home admissions. A majority of nursing home residents are believed to have these disorders, including dementia or other neurological, degenerative illnesses (Jervis and Manson, 2007). Despite the high prevalence of mental disorders in nursing homes and ongoing efforts to improve mental health care as a result of the 1987 Nursing Home Reform Act, the care of nursing home residents with psychiatric disabilities is generally seen as suboptimal. This unacceptable situation is attributed to therapeutic nihilism, inadequate Medicare and Medicaid reimbursement for psychiatric care to nursing homes and physicians, staff orientation mostly toward physical care, and insufficient mental health expertise. Even though formal expertise may be lacking, however, staff often use informal strategies for managing behavioral problems in nursing homes (Jervis and Manson, 2007).

In nursing homes, assistance with activities of daily living (ADLs) is the main source of one-on-one interactions between residents and direct care staff members (Sloane et al., 2007). This case is particularly true for residents who have moderate or severe dementia—those whose impaired cognitive and communication skills often limit participation in group communication and activities. The most concentrated ADL interactions between staff and residents occur during morning care: the period of time between 7:00 AM and 12:00 PM when caregivers are engaged with residents in activities related to bathing, grooming, oral hygiene, dressing, and toileting, which is usually provided during a single, concentrated period of time (Sloane et al., 2007). Morning care of nursing home residents with dementia also presents considerable opportunity for the stimulation of pain and discomfort. Further, not all residents respond favorably to encouragement of independence; it is sometimes too stressful and leads to frustration and agitation.

Positive mood is an integral component of quality of life for nursing home residents who have Alzheimer's disease [(AD) Williams and Tappen, 2007]. Traditional interventions to improve mood, such as cognitive and interpersonal therapies, require communication abilities that may be compromised in individuals who have AD. Yet, maintaining a positive mood in individuals who have advancing AD is important to their already compromised quality of life. Interventions suited to nursing home residents who have AD that would increase positive mood would likely improve the quality of life for those residents.

People who have had a stroke and have eating disorders resulting from a lack of neurological coordination may also have diminished vocal abilities (Quilliam et al., 2001). Those who sustain a stroke and have language impairment (also known as "aphasia") sometimes demonstrate improvement in linguistic skills following intensive speech therapy (Kumlien and Axelsson, 2002). Even though aphasia afflicts more than 30 percent of people who have had a stroke and recover after just a couple months, nearly 60 percent have chronic aphasia (six months or more). Further, people who have had a stroke and have mental impairment may have mood disorders (Kumlien and Axelsson, 2002). Fear of falling, the effects of medications (Vogelsmeier, Scott-Cawiezell, and Zellmer, 2007), illness, and fatigue often result in limited treatments (Williams and Tappen, 2007). All such emotional conditions can bring about various challenges to the resident's psychosocial and personal integrity.

Because aphasia and cognitive dysfunction are so prevalent in these residents (Mitchell et al., 2003; Mackenzie and Lowit, 2007), staff members and speech therapists can also use this time to rehabilitate and enhance resident integrity. It is noteworthy that research on medical interaction shows that patients' communicative behaviors influence those of medical staff caring for them (Street, 2001). Hence, positive interaction exhibited by the residents can reinforce the interpersonal skills of their speech therapists.

Clearly, treating residents who have such cognitive conditions requires a person-centered ("resident-centered" or "patient-centered") approach to care (Breen et al., 2009), especially for morning care. Such resident-centered care would require that a facility's supervisory staff not only permit but also encourage nursing assistants to individualize care (Sloane et al., 2007; Breen et al., 2009). Such care would also require allocating more time to in-room activities and less to having residents congregate in central dining and activity areas. Further, this kind of care would require awareness of and careful assessment for pain and its expression. If activity and nursing staff members could also be involved in aspects of morning care, for some residents, this, too, would enhance the possibility of making morning care more pleasant and resident-centered as well as improve overall quality of life (Sloane et al., 2007; Breen et al., 2009).

The nursing home setting poses particular challenges to pain assessment and treatment (Wu et al., 2005a, 2005b), ranging from the cognitive and communication challenges presented by some nursing home residents to broad and obstructive societal beliefs about aging and pain that may be reflected in staff attitudes about pain management (Clark, Jones, and Pennington, 2004). Inadequate pain assessment and management is a significant issue in many settings, because pain is associated with reduced overall quality of life, depression and anxiety, reduced mobility, impaired sleep or insomnia, delayed healing, poor nutrition, and reduced involvement in recreational activities. Estimates of pain prevalence among nursing home residents are high (Clark, Jones, and Pennington, 2004). About 25 percent to 35 percent of residents report daily pain of moderate to severe intensity. Yet, about 25 percent of nursing home residents with daily pain received no analgesics at all. Experts agree that pain can be ameliorated through a process of formalized pain assessment and the appropriate use of pharmacologic agents and nonpharmacologic interventions.

Finally, behavioral problems in nursing homes are common with prevalence rates ranging from 26 percent to 64 percent (Jervis and Manson, 2007). Requests for psychiatric consultations are usually triggered by behavioral symptoms; many of these behaviors are related to dementia and its associated agitation and aggression. In nursing homes in the United States, social inappropriateness, resisting care, and verbal abuse are the most common behavioral problems (Jervis and Manson, 2007).

Rural Nursing Homes

The logistical underpinnings of the capacity of present-day, rural nursing home service capacity are not yet completely understood. Oftentimes, the availability of providers is interpreted as a fairly accurate gauge of capacity, and in that regard rural nursing homes habitually lag behind urban nursing homes. What lacks clarity is whether supply factors in and of themselves constitute adequate assessments of capacity. In any case, rural nursing homes are starting to increase their acquisitions and development of adult day programs, respite and hospice services (Mor and Allen, 1987), and housing options (Schlenker and Shaughnessy, 1996). Numerous variables—especially limited staffing which is often the case in rural nursing homes—can diminish the capacity to deliver adequate care for failing or imminently terminal residents. There may also be a small threshold regarding the transportation or transfer of rural nursing home residents to specialized hospitals (Shah, Fennell, and Mor, 2001).

This chapter has provided information related to the dimensions and factors that contribute to the variability in the quality of care in nursing home care settings. For example, deficiency citations, the number and types of staff members employed, resident integrity, the overall size of the given nursing home, and the geographical and cultural compositions of nursing homes can all influence the quality of the care they deliver. The next chapter examines policies concerning minimum staffing levels in nursing homes in the United States.

CHAPTER 4

Persistent Citations for the Deficiency of Pressure Ulcers

Pressure ulcers are prevalent in nursing homes, and the quality of life of residents is adversely affected by them (Gorecki et al., 2009). A series of government reports in recent years have revealed concerns about the low quality of care and the high frequency of deficiency citations in nursing homes. The U.S. Department of Health and Human Services (HHS) found that both the percentage of nursing homes with deficiencies and the average number of deficiencies per facility grew between 1998 and 2001 (U.S. Department of Health and Human Services, 2003). More than 91 percent of nursing homes were cited annually by state governments for various deficiencies because of noncompliance with federal quality standards between 2005 and 2007 (U.S. Department of Health and Human Services, 2008). The General Accounting Office (GAO) also noticed that about 40 percent of the homes had persistent serious deficiencies in a sequence of government inspections (U.S. General Accounting Office, 1999). If the presence of isolated deficiencies is related to chance, then persistent deficiencies reflect long-term insensitivity to or inability to correct identified problems—more harmful than isolated deficiencies to vulnerable elderly and disabled residents in nursing homes. Identifying factors associated with persistent deficiency citations in nursing homes is important in developing solutions to improve quality of nursing home care and resident safety. Of the 185 deficiency items cited, we examined the risk factors associated with the top-ranked deficiency—pressure ulcers—in relation to nursing home care (see table 4.1).

Pressure ulcers are a common but preventable and treatable medical problem in nursing homes. Between 17 percent and 35 percent of residents have pressure ulcers on admission to nursing facilities (Smith, 1995). Despite being considered a localized soft-tissue wound, pressure ulcers can cause serious clinical complications and a negative social impact on residents, including local infection, sepsis, osteomyelitis, substantially increased mortality rate and increases in nursing care time, cost, and adverse events (Kuhn and Coulter, 1992; Smith, 1995). The cost of treating pressure ulcers in the United States could be as high as $11 billion per year (Reddy, Gill, and Rochon, 2006). As shown in table 4.1, pressure ulcers represent the most frequently cited medical deficiency in the 11 years from 1997 to 2007. They are also one of the key indicators listed under "Nursing Home Compare" on the Centers for Medicare and Medicaid Services (CMS) website, a unique resident decision-making tool for the public to judge and choose nursing homes based on their performance (Centers for Medicare and Medicaid Services, 2009a). Identifying the risk factors and providing evidence-based knowledge related to persistent deficiencies in treating pressure ulcers should be priorities for reducing their number as well as in preventing resident deficiencies from resurfacing in nursing homes. Although numerous studies have discussed risk factors for pressure ulcers and related deficiencies in nursing homes, to our knowledge, few studies have examined their development from organizational, management, aggregate residential, and market factor perspectives.

Deficiencies such as deficiencies in management, resident rights, food sanitation, and pharmacy have become important measures of nursing home quality because they reflect the process aspects of performance. State governments survey nursing homes under contract with CMS annually at 9- to 15-month intervals to inspect their compliance with federal quality standards. The protocol of these state surveys on pressure ulcer treatment also focuses on examining process measures, such as prevention and treatment—comprehensive assessment, comprehensive care planning, and nutrition.

Persistent citations for deficiency indicate a managerial failure that is probably avoidable if care processes are carefully assessed and followed. The Resident Assessment Protocols (RAPs) mandated by the 1987 Omnibus Budget Reconciliation Act (OBRA) clearly demonstrate the process for evaluation of clinically avoidable ulcers and adequate treatment. Resident assessment/reassessment and care planning have become routines that are performed quarterly in nursing homes. Literature also supports that care processes, including resident assessment and care planning, are positively associated with the nursing home quality (Morris et al., 2002; Wipke-Tevis et al., 2004; Dellefield, 2006; Lee et al., 2009). Comprehensive resident assessment is critical for identifying prolonged pressure, sensory loss, immobility, malnutrition and the need for repositioning and pressure-reducing bed support. Comprehensive/interdisciplinary care planning

Table 4.1 The Top Twenty Deficiencies in U.S. Nursing Homes, 1997–2007

Variable	Average number of deficiencies per year	Description
F371	3,694	Food sanitation
F309	3,030	Highest practicable care
F323	2,707	Hazard-free environment
F281	2,326	Professional standards
F279	2,195	Comprehensive care plan
F253	2,191	Housekeeping
F314[a]	2,149	Pressure ulcers
F324	2,074	Accident prevention
F241	2,052	Dignity
F441	1,655	Infection control
F514	1,636	Records complete
F272	1,635	Comprehensive assessments
F329	1,588	Drugs
F312	1,532	ADL services
F221	1,372	Physical restraints
F225	1,266	Criminal staff/abuse
F282	1,246	Assessment by qualified staff
F465	1,214	Other environment
F246	1,174	Accommodate needs
F332	1,134	Medication errors >5%

Note: The average number of deficiencies per year comes from authors' calculations. ADL= Activity of daily living
[a]Top one ranked deficiency related to medical care.

and its implementation, including incontinence care to keep residents' skin clean and dry, repositioning, nutritional interventions, pressure-relieving devices, and therapeutic treatments would prevent pressure ulcers from developing and accelerate the healing process (Smith, 1995). Thus, nursing home–derived pressure ulcers and persistent problems in preventing and treating pressure ulcers should not emerge as deficiencies if care processes are in place. Therefore, we hypothesize that comprehensive resident assessment and care planning is associated with fewer persistent deficiencies in treating pressure ulcers, controlling for other organizational, residential, and market factors.

Another important factor related to deficiencies of treatment of pressure ulcers is nurse staffing. A series of studies has found higher nurse staffing levels are associated with a lower prevalence rate of pressures ulcers (Castle, 2003b; Zhang and Grabowski, 2004), a lower incidence rate of pressure ulcers (Grabowski and Angelelli, 2004; Wan, Zhang, and Unruh, 2006; Zhang et al., 2006), and a lower number of total deficiencies that include pressure ulcers (Harrington et al., 2000b; Konetzka et al., 2004; Zhang, Unruh, and Wan, 2008). A higher total number of nursing staff was found to be associated with lower risk-adjusted pressure ulcer prevalence and fewer deficiency citations, based on a study using a sample of 897 California nursing homes (Dellefield, 2006). Care of pressure ulcers requires interdisciplinary teamwork (Berlowitz et al., 2003) and intensive labor (Schnelle et al., 2004b) in addition to good management. An adequate and stable nurse workforce ensures lower pressure ulcer prevalence and fewer numbers of deficiencies (Park and Stearns, 2009). Conversely, without adequate and stable nurse staffing, persistent deficiencies are more likely to occur. Thus, we hypothesized that a higher number of nurse staff is associated with a lower likelihood of persistent deficiencies, controlling for other organizational, residential, and market factors.

Methods

Analytical Plan

To examine persistent deficiencies in nursing homes, we used a pooled cross-sectional analysis for all nursing homes in the United States certified by Medicare or Medicaid or dually certified by Medicare and Medicaid from 1997 to 2007. Each nursing home has multiple observations of deficiencies over time in a pooled cross-sectional design, which is better than a longitudinal design to capture the count of consecutive years of deficiency citations for each nursing home. Theoretically, in 11 years of observation, a nursing home could have from 0 to 10 consecutive years of deficiency citations. The pooled cross-sectional design also provided the opportunity to include analysis of nursing homes that would otherwise be excluded in panel data analysis.

Sources of Data

The data used to test the proposed hypotheses include Online Survey Certification and Reporting (OSCAR) data and Area Resource File (ARF) data. OSCAR contains nursing home deficiency citation information that state surveyors collect during annual inspections following CMS standards. The state inspections take place once a year within a 9- to 15-month interval and represent a snapshot of nursing home quality during the few days of inspections. A citation is given if a nursing home is found to be noncompliant with the minimum CMS standard in any of the 185 inspection items. If a deficiency is not corrected, it does not exclude the possibility that the same deficiency is cited in the following inspection. CMS monetarily punishes nursing homes that receive life-threatening and persistent deficiencies. The CMS "Special Focus Facility Initiative" is another effort to help nursing homes improve their performance (Centers for Medicare and Medicaid Services, 2009b). At this time, OSCAR is an authoritative source for providing nursing home deficiency information and the most comprehensive repository of nurse staffing, organizational, and aggregate resident data of nursing homes. OSCAR data have been widely used to measure nursing home care process, staffing, and quality in government reports (U.S. Department of Health and Human Services, 2008; U.S. General Accounting Office, 2008), media (Duhigg, 2007) and research (Castle and Engberg, 2007a; Harrington, Swan, and Carillo, 2007; Grabowski and Stevenson, 2008).

The market factors potentially influencing persistent nursing home deficiencies were acquired from the ARF 2000, which was developed by the U.S. Bureau of Health Professions. Eleven years of OSCAR data were merged based on provider ID (identification) to develop a workable data set that excludes new or closed nursing homes during the study period.

Once all study variables were identified in their respective databases, we cleaned the data to eliminate extreme outliers and potentially erroneous values before further analysis. This study adopted the data-cleaning criteria developed by CMS. Facilities were excluded from our analysis if they presented: (1) more residents than beds; (2) no RN (registered nurse) hours and had 60 or more beds (because federal regulations require facilities with 60 or more beds to have an RN on duty for 8 hours a day, 7 days a week); (3) more than 12 total hours per resident day and less than 0.5 total hours per resident day; or (4) zero residents (Harrington et al., 2000b; Berlowitz et al., 2003; Konetzka et al., 2004; Schnelle et al., 2004b; Zhang, Unruh, and Wan, 2008; Park and Stearns, 2009). Facilities in Puerto Rico, the U.S. territories, and Washington, D.C., were excluded from analysis because of the small number of OSCAR surveys from these locations (Harrington et al., 2000b; Intrator et al., 2005; Mueller et al., 2006). If facility data had duplicate identifiers, we used the most recent survey data; if the dates of the surveys were identical, we randomly selected one (Castle, 2001). The original OSCAR data contained surveys of 12,689 nursing homes. After data cleaning, 11,176 nursing homes remained in the study, which represented 88 percent of the original number of nursing homes.

Measurements

Dependent Variable. The dependent variable in this study is the persistent deficiency of pressure ulcers cited by state surveyors at each nursing home across the 11 years from 1997 to 2007. Theoretically, the deficiency of pressure ulcer could repeat itself from 2 to 11 years with or without intervals in our study. The persistency of pressure ulcer deficiency is defined as a dummy variable coded as 0 and 1, where 1 represents two or more consecutive years of pressure ulcer deficiency for a specific nursing home during the 11 years while 0 indicates that there is only an isolated stand-alone deficiency or the nursing home has no deficiencies.

Independent Variables. To test the two hypotheses, we examined three independent variables in association with the persistent deficiencies of pressure ulcers: comprehensive resident assessment, comprehensive care planning, and total nurse staffing. The first two independent variables were measured negatively by examining the deficiency citations given for noncompliance with the care process standards. Zero (0) represents no deficiency and 1 represents one or more deficiency citations.

Total nurse staffing was measured by the hours per resident day for the total number of nurses, which included registered nurses, licensed practice nurses, and nurse aids. All full-time, part-time, and contract nurses were included. The original nurse staffing measures from the OSCAR data were treated as full-time equivalent (FTE). To be consistent and comparable with CMS and other studies, we transferred the FTE to hours per resident day by computing FTE × 70/14/(number of residents) because one FTE in OSCAR is defined as 70 hours of work in 14 days (Zhang and Grabowski, 2004; Zhang et al., 2006).

Covariates. The control variables in this study included organizational, management, aggregate residential, and market variables that are theoretically or empirically associated with the persistent deficiencies of pressure ulcers. Organizational variables included size of facility, ownership, chain membership, hospital affiliation, percentage of Medicaid recipients, total nurse staffing, and occupancy rate. Management variables included the existence of a quality assurance (QA) committee, QA committee meetings/recommendations, nutrition and nutritional adequacy. Size was measured as the total number of residents at the time of the survey. Nursing home ownership (for-profit, nonprofit, and government), chain membership, and hospital affiliation were categorical variables. The percentage of Medicaid recipients reflected the proportion of residents receiving Medicaid payment. Occupancy rate was the total number of residents divided by the total number of beds. The Medicaid reimbursement rate was adopted from a study published by Grabowski and a research team at Brown University (Grabowski et al., 2004). The existence of a QA committee, QA committee meetings/recommendations, a comprehensive care plan, nutrition and nutritional adequacy were deficiency measures in which 0 represents no deficiency and 1 represents at least one deficiency cited over 11 years.

Aggregate residential factors include aggregate residential functional status, clinical characteristics, and known risk factors for the development of pressure ulcers, including resident acuity index, number of residents who develop pressure ulcers, skin prevention and number of residents who are bedfast all or most of the time, in a chair all or most of the time, independently ambulatory, ambulatory with assistance or an assistive device, physically restrained, incontinent of bowel, and having dementia.

Market variables include market competition and market demand. Market competition was measured by the Herfindahl-Hirschman (H-H) Index and calculated as:

$$\text{H-H index} = \sum_{i=0}^{n} \frac{(\text{number of beds in a nursing home}}{\text{total number of beds in a county})}$$

(U.S. Department of Health and Human Services, 2008), where i is the number of nursing homes in a county. A higher H-H score indicates less competition. Market demand was measured by the percentage of people 75 years or older in the county where a nursing home is located.

Statistical Analysis

To test the hypotheses and estimate the impact of the three independent variables while controlling the relevant covariates, we proposed a regression model. As the dependent variable—persistent deficiency of pressure ulcers—is a dichotomous categorical variable, we used a binary logistic regression model. Despite 11 years of observations, no time effect was involved because the study applied a pooled cross-sectional design. We used the Hosmer and Lemeshow goodness-of-fit test to evaluate the performance of the model. We used odds ratios and their statistical significances to assess the impact of the hypothesized variables. If an odds ratio is greater than 1, it indicates a positive relationship between the independent variables and the dependent variable. On the other hand, if an odds ratio is less than 1, it indicates a negative relationship. The statistically significant level we examined was fixed at 0.05 and the model results were produced by using SAS 9 [(Cary, NC; version 9.0) computer software].

Results

The results of descriptive analysis are shown in table 4.2. In the 11 years from 1997 to 2007, approximately one third (33.24%) of nursing homes in the nation had persistent deficiencies of pressure ulcers for at least two consecutive years. The number of hours per resident day of total nurse staffing averaged 3.345. There were considerable percentages of nursing homes receiving deficiencies on comprehensive care planning (73.48%) and resident assessment (62.92%).

The results of the logistic regression model of persistent deficiencies of pressure ulcers are illustrated in table 4.3. The Hosmer and Lemeshow Goodness-of-Fit test (Chi-square test) shows that the p value is greater than the 0.05 significance level, which indicates that the model fits the studied data well. The odds ratios of independent variables and their 95 percent confidence intervals (CI) are presented in the table. Comprehensive care planning and resident assessment, two independent variables in hypothesis one, were found to be statistically significant. The odds ratios are 0.669 with a 95 percent CI of (0.603, 0.742) and 0.634 with a 95 percent CI of (0.578, 0.694), which indicates a negative relationship between these two independent variables and the dependent variable. Because the dependent variable, persistent deficiencies of pressure ulcers, was coded as 1, the results suggest that nursing homes with appropriate comprehensive care planning or resident assessment have 33.1 percent and 36.7 percent smaller odds of developing persistent deficiencies of pressure ulcers than those without or with defective comprehensive care planning or resident assessment. Therefore, hypothesis one is supported in this study.

The total number of nursing staff members turns out to be statistically significant in the model as well. Its odds ratio is 0.869 with a 95 percent CI of (0.829, 0.910). The results suggest that nursing homes with a higher total number of nurses have 13.1 percent lower odds of having persistent deficiencies of pressure ulcers. Therefore, hypothesis two is also supported in this study.

The strongest factor associated with a lower chance of developing persistent

Table 4.2 Descriptive Statistics of Study Variables
(N = 11,176)

Variable			
Dependent variable	*Percentage*		
Persistent deficiency			
No persistent deficiency on pressure ulcer	66.76		
Persistent deficiency on pressure ulcer	33.24		
Independent variable (categorical)			
Comprehensive care plan			
No deficiency in 11 years	26.52		
At least one deficiency in 11 years	73.48		
Comprehensive assessment			
No deficiency in 11 years	37.08		
At least one deficiency in 11 years	62.92		
Independent variable (continuous)	*Mean (Std.)*	*Min*	*Max*
Total nurse staffing (per resident per day)	3.345 (1.257)	1.045	11.970
Covariate (categorical)	*Percentage*		
Chain membership			
Chain	57.96		
Not chain	42.04		
Ownership			
For-profit ownership	66.03		
Nonprofit ownership	27.90		
Government ownership	6.07		
Hospital Affiliation			
Hospital-based	8.51		
Not hospital based	91.49		
QA Committee			
No deficiency in 11 years	88.77		
At least one deficiency in 11 years	11.23		
QA Committee meets/plans			
No deficiency in 11 years	88.46		
At least one deficiency in 11 years	11.54		
Nutrition			
No deficiency in 11 years	51.21		
At least one deficiency in 11 years	48.79		
Menus/nutritional adequacy 0 (vs. 1)			
No deficiency in 11 years	67.74		
At least one deficiency in 11 years	32.26		
Covariate (continuous)	*Mean (Std.)*	*Min*	*Max*
Facility size (total number of beds)	115.580 (71.083)	8	1229.550
Occupancy rate	0.849 (0.128)	0.031	1.000
% of Medicaid residents	62.962 (20.645)	0	100.000

Table 4.2 *Continued*
(N = 11,176)

Variable			
Covariate (continuous)	*Mean (Std.)*	*Min*	*Max*
Number of pressure ulcers	6.836 (5.593)	0	75.182
Number of skin preventions	64.375 (43.985)	0	656.364
Bedfast all or most of time	4.832 (5.730)	0	106.727
Independently ambulatory	14.364 (15.259)	0	249.181
Ambulation with assistance or assistive device	30.471 (21.000)	0	518.818
Physically restrained	9.246 (9.472)	0	213.455
Incontinent of bowel	44.450 (34.054)	0	568.364
Dementia	44.159 (31.549)	0	577.909
Acuity index	10.211 (1.292)	3.667	21.058
Market competition	0.202 (0.235)	0.004	1.000
Market demand	0.066 (0.022)	0.013	1.000
Medicaid reimbursement rate	110.301 (20.836)	74	165.510

Note: Std. = standard deviation

deficiencies of pressure ulcers in this study is market demand. Market demand has an odds ratio of 0.015, which indicates that higher market demand is associated with lower probability of developing persistent deficiencies of pressure ulcers. The strongest risk factors associated with a greater chance of developing persistent deficiencies of pressure ulcers in this study is chain affiliation. Chain-affiliated nursing homes have a 19.5 percent greater chance of developing persistent deficiencies of pressure ulcers.

As expected, all variables (such as existence of a quality assurance/improvement committee) related to better management of pressure ulcers were negatively associated with a lower likelihood of developing persistent deficiencies of pressure ulcers. Some variables (such as number of residents with pressure ulcers) considered as resident risk factors correlated with a higher likelihood of developing persistent deficiencies of pressure ulcers. Surprisingly, five other commonly identified resident risk factors were not found to be statistically significant in this model. Both the percentage of Medicaid recipients and state Medicaid reimbursement were positively associated with higher likelihood of developing persistent deficiencies of pressure ulcers. With an odds ratio of 0.771, market competition was found to be negatively associated with the development of persistent deficiencies of pressure ulcers.

Table 4.3 Results of Binary Logistic Regression of Persistent Deficiencies

Variable	Odds ratio (95% CI)
Independent	
Comprehensive care plan 0 (vs. 1)	0.669 (0.603, 0.742)*
Comprehensive assessment 0 (vs. 1)	0.634 (0.578, 0.694)*
Total nurse staffing	0.886 (0.827, 0.908)*
Covariate	
Nonprofit (versus for-profit)	0.945 (0.848, 1.054)
Government (versus for-profit)	1.083 (0.880, 1.334)
Chain affiliation Yes (vs. no)	1.195 (1.090, 1.311)*
Hospital-based Yes (vs. no)	1.056 (0.871, 1.280)
QA Committee 0 (vs. 1)	0.809 (0.711, 0.921)*
QA Committee meets/recommends 0 (vs.1)	0.756 (0.667, 0.857)*
Nutrition 0 (vs. 1)	0.571 (0.525, 0.622)*
Menus/nutritional adequacy 0 (vs. 1)	0.753 (0.689, 0.824)*
Continuous Variables	
Facility size (Total number of beds)	1.000 (0.999, 1.002)
Occupancy rate	0.341 (0.213, 0.546)*
% of Medicaid residents	1.004 (1.002, 1.007)*
Pressure sores	1.052 (1.037, 1.067)*
Number of skin preventions	1.003 (1.001, 1.005)*
Bedfast all or most of time	0.999 (0.989, 1.009)
Independently ambulatory	0.995 (0.990, 0.999)*
Ambulation with assistance or assistive device	1.005 (1.001, 1.009)*
Physically restrained	1.003 (0.997, 1.008)
Incontinent of bowel	0.992 (0.988, 0.996)*
Dementia	1.000 (0.997, 1.004)
Acuity index	1.002 (0.952, 1.054)
Market competition	0.771 (0.630, 0.945)*
Market demand	0.015 (0.002, 1.121)*
Medicaid reimbursement rate	1.005 (1.003, 1.008)*

Hosmer and Lemeshow goodness-of-fit tests
Chi-square (df = 9.351 (8)
p-value = 0.314

Note: Skin prevention = # of Skin preventions /100; CI = Confidence Interval; df = degree of freedom
  * statistically significant at $p < 0.05$ level.

Discussion

The clinical risk factors of stand-alone pressure ulcers have been identified since the evidence-based clinical practice guidelines published by the Agency for Health Care Policy and Research in 1992 (U.S. Department of Health and Human Services, 1992). The organizational risk factors of stand-alone pressure ulcer deficiencies in nursing homes have also been well studied (Aaronson, Zinn, and Rosko, 1994; Dellefield, 2006). This study expanded prior research and provides insight into risk factors associated with persistent deficiencies of pressure ulcers in nursing homes from 1997 to 2007. The results of this study indicate that in addition to clinical factors, organizational, management, and market risk factors are associated with the development of persistent deficiencies of pressure ulcers.

This study was motivated by the CMS "Special Focus Facility" (SFF) initiative published in recent years as a way to identify a history of persistent serious quality problems and stimulate improvements of quality of care (Centers for Medicare and Medicaid Services, 2009b). Although we did not follow the SFF methodology exactly to identify "special" nursing homes, our approach investigated the persistence of nursing home deficiencies in a broader sense that allowed us to include all persistent deficiencies of pressure ulcers in the study. This study expanded the SFF approaches in identifying poor performers for public reference in choosing nursing homes and discovered risk factors for potential interventions.

Total nurse staffing, comprehensive care planning, and resident assessment were found to be effective structural and process improvements for better quality of care. On one hand, our findings support the theoretical relationship between structure, process, and performance. On the other hand, we believe that the organizational structure and process factors, including the presence of a QA committee and QA committee meetings/recommendations, are potential interventions nursing homes should consider and implement appropriately. This finding is consistent with those of Castle (2002), who found that higher nurse staffing is associated with fewer persistent deficiencies in nursing homes, and Berlowitz and Frantz (2007) who found that process factors related to quality improvement are effective in reducing pressure ulcers (Castle and Fogel, 2002; Berlowitz and Frantz, 2007).

Market factors, including market demand and market competition, were strong indicators of fewer persistent deficiencies of pressure ulcers. The nursing home industry has been highly regulated for years. Sustained nursing home deficiencies necessitate the exploration of alternative strategies to improve outcomes. Both the CMS "Nursing Home Compare" public website and SFF are governmental efforts to maneuver government and market mechanisms simultaneously because they stimulate nursing home market competition on quality by publicizing information on nursing home performance.

One of the limitations of this study is the fact that although we computed years of consecutive deficiency citations, clinical severity of deficiency was not considered in the analysis. We do not think the same deficiency should resurface once it is cited regardless of its severity because (1) there are multiple, evidence-based clinical practice guidelines, (2) pressure ulcers are a preventable and treatable disease, and (3) the deficiency citations document inappropriate process or treatment that did not follow current accepted practice guidelines. A second limitation of this study is that although the deficiencies reported in the OSCAR database represent the best and most official deficiency data available, state and surveyor variations in issuing citations have created reliability and comparability issues in deficiency analysis (U.S. General Accounting Office, 2005). An additional limitation is the fact that the organizational/management factors are measured by deficiency citations that are proxy measures in the secondary database. Finally, it should be emphasized that our study focuses on only pressure ulcers. It may have implications for correcting persistent deficiencies for other clinical measures, such as urinary tract infections, falls, and physical restraints and pain management in nursing homes, but we caution generalization.

Persistent deficiencies are a serious challenge for improving quality in nursing homes, and persistent deficiencies of pressure ulcers have been a sustained and endemic problem. Our study shows that a multidisciplinary approach integrating clinical, organizational, management, and market strategies provides better interventions for persistent deficiencies, and we suggest the effectiveness of the multidisciplinary intervention on other deficiency citations be examined in future studies.

CHAPTER 5

Factors Influencing Residents' Outcomes

Research on the determinants and consequences of poor quality of nursing home care has focused on the regulatory impact and policy constraints such as minimum staffing requirements, workforce interventions, staff training, and licensing. Concerted efforts have been made to improve care through the development of prospective payments or incentive payments for innovative services. However, long-term care research has generated inconclusive results (Schnelle, Newman, and Fogarty, 1990a, 1990b; Rantz et al., 2001; Mor et al., 2009). Because a limited number of evidence-based or empirical research studies have been conducted using longitudinal study designs and panel analysis of nursing home data, the underlying causal mechanisms associated with poor quality of nursing home care have not thoroughly been explored. Without specifications of causal factors influencing nursing home quality, it is impossible to formulate successful policies to improve quality of care and resident outcomes. Better understanding of the relationships of key contextual and facility factors with nurse staffing, nursing care quality, and rehabilitative care could lead to the development of appropriate intervention strategies for quality improvement in nursing homes.

This chapter examines how key nursing home contextual, organizational (staffing) and process (nursing care adequacy and rehabilitation) factors influence resident outcomes. Research questions are (1) What factors are associated with the improvement of resident outcomes? (2) Can previous levels of quality influence later levels of quality? (3) Do time-specific measures of nursing influence the improvement of resident outcomes when lagged effects of quality and contextual factors are considered? Using a panel of nursing homes with autoregressive latent trajectory modeling, we assessed the relationships of staffing, nursing care adequacy, and rehabilitative care to each wave of quality improvement, holding constant facility and contextual factors in the investigation of individual change trajectories. While controlling for facility and contextual factors, we hypothesized that nursing homes with higher nurse staffing, more rehabilitative care, and greater nursing care adequacy show improved resident outcomes.

A Systems Framework for Research in Nursing Homes

Donabedian's structure-process-outcome (SPO) model has been widely used in nursing home studies to depict relationships between structure (staff to resident ratios and skill mix, physical properties of a facility, or policies and procedures), process (care activities) and outcome factors (health status and consequences of care) (Donabedian, 1966). This familiar model, however, fails to account for the dynamic nature of facilities and the influence of internal and external forces affecting nursing care quality and resident outcomes. Much of the research has examined the linkages between only two components (i.e., structure and outcomes). No studies have systematically examined the relationship of structural and process components to resident outcomes, using a longitudinal study. Goodson, Jang, and Rantz (2008) noted that the overall quality of nursing home care can be assessed by aggregating various quality domains, such as structure, process and outcome aspects of care, from a Bayesian network approach. Further, the relationships between the change trajectories of resident outcomes and their determinants should be explored.

Unruh and Wan (2004) expanded the SPO framework to postulate that the functioning of health care institutions is contextually influenced by external environment influences such as the socioeconomic and demographic characteristics of the population, and state, metropolitan, and rural/urban location characteristics (e.g., market forces or enforcement of regulations). Structural components are the facility's physical and human resources, and other characteristics such as bed size, ownership, chain affiliation, and payment mix. Staffing is depicted as a separate structural component because of its association with other structural variables (e.g., for-profit homes and lower staffing levels) and interaction with processes of care [e.g., numbers of RNs (registered nurses) and lower use of restraints]. Process refers to both clinical and nonclinical services, as well as staff communication when assessing, planning, and delivering care. Examples of resident outcomes include measures of physical functioning, continence, and freedom from pressure ulcers.

Related Research

Nurse Staffing, Nursing Care Process, and Quality

The positive relationship between nurse staffing levels and the quality of nursing home care has been widely demonstrated (Cohen and Spector, 1996; Bliesmer et al., 1998; Castle and Fogel, 1998; Porell et al., 1998; Harrington et al., 2000b; Wan, 2003; Schnelle et al., 2004a; Unruh and Wan, 2004; Seblega et al., 2009). Studies have associated greater RN or licensed nurses hours per resident day with better care (Shnelle et al., 2004b), lower levels of deficiency citations (Harrington et al., 2000b), a higher probability of discharge home, a lower probability of death (Bliesmer et al., 1998), fewer pressure ulcers, better mental and functional status of residents (Cohen and Spector, 1996; Porell et al., 1998), and lower use of restraints (Castle and Fogel, 1998).

State survey reports and research have begun to indicate that inadequate nursing care *processes* lead to poor resident outcomes. Processes such as failure to provide comprehensive care plans for residents and poor resident assessment remain among the top 10 deficiencies cited by state surveyors (Harrington et al., 2000b). Braun (1991) found that nursing processes, such as positioning, catheter care, personal hygiene, and lower mortality increased the likelihood of discharge among VA (Veterans Affairs) nursing home residents. In another study, facilities that have higher catheter use, less skin care, and low resident participation in organized activities tend to have negative resident outcomes (Spector and Takada, 1991).

Nursing care quality was measured by multiple indicators of nursing home structure, process, and outcomes of care using annual assessments of nursing home deficiencies made by state agency surveyors (Wan, 2003). A one-factor or unidimensional measurement model for each of two quality constructs was confirmed by the data in each study year. This empirical study of the relationship between adequate levels of nursing care and nursing care quality demonstrates that a positive relationship exists between the process and outcome dimensions of the quality of nursing care.

Contextual and Facility Characteristics and Quality

Legislation or Reimbursement Policies. An external environmental factor may influence nursing home performance and quality through its impact on structural variables. The Balanced Budget Act (BBA) of 1997, which initiated a prospective payment system for Medicare reimbursement to nursing homes, sub-stantially reduced Medicare payments to nursing homes (Gage, 1999). Unruh, Zhang, and Wan (2006) found that the BBA had a negative effect on both nurse staffing and resident outcomes. However, the 1999 Balanced Budget Reconcilia-tion Act (BBRA) and the 2000 Benefits Improvement and Protection Act (BIPA), both of which attempted to soften the effect of the BBA, had positive effects on both staffing and outcomes.

Characteristics of the Facility. Bed size, ownership, chain affiliation, payment mix, and average acuity level of residents are considered to be important orga-nizational factors influencing nursing care and quality in nursing homes. John-son et al. (2004) report that small, nonprofit, and non-chain-affiliated facilities have fewer lawsuits brought against them (a proxy for poor quality) and that a higher incident of lawsuits is positively associated with deficiency citations. Bed size has been positively associated with the use of physical restraints (Cas-tle, 2000).

Other research has found that for-profit facilities have fewer professional nurses (Greene and Monahan, 1981; Harrington et al., 2001), provide lower quality of services (Chou, 2002), and receive more federal deficiency citations (Harrington and Millman, 2001) than nonprofit facilities. Because two thirds of nursing homes in the United States are for-profit (Harrington et al., 2001), this is a major concern. Resident acuity is important to the analysis because rising acuity levels of residents requires more extensive and intensive interventions (Rantz et al., 1999a). Finally, a recent study on the relationship between pro-vider performance and activity of daily living (ADL) change shows that the degree to which a quality indicator (such as ADL change) may be affected by provider performance varies by resident characteristics (Phillips et al., 2008). Thus, the development of pay-for-performance should pay greater attention to individual characteristics as well as contextual variables that may influence resident outcomes.

Characteristics of the Market or Environment. Regional location, metropolitan size, and the percentage of elderly individuals (75 years of age or older) in the population are pertinent contextual variables for explaining the variation in nursing home quality. Gessert and Calkins (2001) found that the more concen-trated the older population, the greater is the use of feeding tubes. Coburn, Bolda, and Keith (2003) found higher rates of nursing home use among rural residents.

Competition, driven by the rising demand for nursing home care due to the increase in the elderly population and the stringency in the certificate-of-need (CON) regulation, may lead to worsening of the quality of nursing home care (Nyman, 1988, 1989). Because age composition of the geographic area influences the supply of and demand for nursing home beds, studies of nursing home quality should incorporate the percentage of elderly people as a control variable.

Methods

This study explores how nurse staffing (NS), rehabilitation (REHAB), and nursing care deficiency citations (NCD) influence resident outcomes when the effects of contextual and other structural factors are simultaneously considered. It investigates the net influence of nursing care factors on the improvement of resident outcomes in seven consecutive years (1997–2003), controlling for nursing home characteristics. We hypothesize that nurse staffing and rehabilitation services have a positive effect on quality, while nursing care deficiencies have a negative effect. These predictors are considered to vary over time in relationship to quality, whereas several control variables, such as facility and market characteristics, are constant over time.

Sources of Data

This study uses OSCAR data from fiscal years 1997 to 2003. The data include state inspector survey information (collected every 9 to 15 months) to verify nursing home compliance with regulatory requirements and facility self-report on resident conditions. OSCAR contains three areas of information: (1) characteristics of the facility, (2) resident census and conditions, and (3) deficiency measurements.

To eliminate extreme outliers, we excluded facilities with: (1) 15 or fewer residents (Harrington et al., 2000b); (2) total hours per resident day <0.5 or >12 (Konetzka et al., 2004); and (3) nursing staffing beyond mean ± 2 standard deviations. After cleaning, the study included 11,197 nursing homes.

Measures

Quality Index. This study develops a quality index from nursing home self-reported measures of quality in OSCAR database. Self-reported measures are selected resident conditions reported by nursing homes that have been used in prior studies (Zhang and Grabowski, 2004). The measures are the incidence of pressure ulcers, physical restraints, and indwelling catheters. These measures represent three important aspects of resident outcomes: skin integrity, mobility, and bowel/bladder status. They have been shown to be negatively associated with nurse staffing and rehabilitation in prior studies. An annual rate of each of these was calculated as follows: (number of residents with conditions present on admission − number of residents with the conditions)/total residents. The three measures were then integrated into one quality index (QI) by using principal component analysis to assign separate weights for each of the quality indicators. The weights for incidence rates of indwelling catheters, physical restraints, and pressure ulcers were 0.670, 0.695, and 0.741, respectively, with a 49.35 percent sum of squared loadings. The QI was formed by multiplying the negative value of the facility's incidence rate times the principal component weight for each type of incident, then summing all three up. This index represents the facility's quality—the higher the index, the higher the quality.

Nurse Staffing. To be consistent with nurse staffing measures in the literature, full-time equivalent (FTE) of nurse staffing in OSCAR data were transformed to hours per resident day, as follows: nursing FTE × 70/14/number of total residents. OSCAR FTEs include full-time, part-time, and contract nurses. The nurse staffing (NS) variable is the sum of RN, LPN/LVN, and nurse aide hours per resident day.

Nursing Care Deficiency/Adequacy. The total number of federal citations of deficiencies in nursing care, made annually by surveyors, is a measure of the adequacy of nursing care. Of the many deficiencies measured, we selected ones associated with the nursing care process: assessment (F272–F278 variables in the OSCAR data file), care plan development (F279), care plan requirements (F280), sufficient nursing care (F353), training (F497), and competency (F498). These F-tags were summed up to a nursing care adequacy/deficiency (NCD) index. The higher the index value, the poorer the nursing care adequacy.

Use of Rehabilitative Services. OSCAR data capture the total number of rehabilitative services (physical therapy, occupational therapy, and speech therapy). From this, we computed a rate of rehabilitation services (REH) per 100 residents per year per nursing home.

Time-Constant or Time-Invariant Predictor Variables. The eight covariates measured in 1997 used as control variables are: (1) bed size, (2) private ownership, (3) chain affiliation, (4) average acuity level, (5) percentage of Medicare recipients, (6) southern region, (7) rural/urban location, and (8) percentage of those individuals 75 years or older in the area where the facility is located. Bed size, average acuity index, percentage of Medicare and percentage of individuals 75 years or older in the area are continuous variables. The rest are dichotomous variables.

We use an acuity index based on nursing home self-reported resident data—a combination of an ADL index and a special treatments index. It is the sum of the proportion of residents with certain characteristics times their associated weights, as follows: proportion of residents [totally dependent for eating × 3] + [requiring the assistance of staff with eating × 2] + [independent or requiring supervision eating] + [totally dependent of toileting × 5] + [requiring the assistance of staff with toileting × 3] + [independent or requiring supervision with toileting] + [totally dependent for transferring × 5] + [requiring the assistance of staff with transferring × 3] + [independent or requiring supervision for transferring × 1] + [bedfast × 5] + [chairbound × 3] + [ambulatory] (Cowles Research Group, 2005). The special treatments index is the sum of the proportions of residents receiving respiratory care, suctioning, intravenous therapy, tracheostomy care, and parenteral feeding. The values of the ADL and the special treatments indices are then summed. The range of the final acuity index is from 3 to 23.

Analytical Design and Approach

A panel study design was formulated to observe nursing home quality in 1997 and in six consecutive years (1998–2003). The seven waves of nursing home data enable us to investigate the influence of both time-constant and time-varying specific predictor variables on the change trajectories of resident outcomes or quality. In addition, the lagged effect of quality in the analysis can be considered. Because this investigation focuses on individual trajectories and the effect of earlier values in determining the level of repeated measures in quality, we adopt the autoregressive latent trajectory (ALT) modeling approach, proposed by Bollen and Curran (2004). This approach expands latent growth curve modeling of nursing home quality with an autoregressive endogenous variable (e.g., the repeated QI measures). This specific growth curve model is used for five reasons: (1) the relationships between multiple causes and outcomes of nursing home care cannot be adequately explained by conventional regression methods; (2) the means, variances, and covariances of repeated measures of continuous variables can be investigated; (3) random coefficients are used to capture individual facility differences in the initial observation period and the growth trend; (4) both time-invariant and time-varying covariates can be included as predictors or control variables for an endogenous variable; and (5) the change patterns of QI over the time span of seven years can be delineated so that we can test the concomitant effects of the three time-specific/time-varying variables such as nurse staffing, rehabilitative service use, and nursing care adequacy on the quality index in each wave. The colinearity of these predictor variables was investigated; the highest intercorrelation was observed between nurse staffing and rehabilitation service use in 2002, with a coefficient of 0.284.

Initially, without including any control or predictor variables, a single-indicator growth curve model with autoregressed QI measures was formulated to include a measure of QI97 at Time 0, an intercept (initial level), and a slope (growth trend) factor. QI97 was treated as a predetermined predictor of the repeated measure so it could be included in the model to detect its lagged effect. These three component factors are assumed to be correlated in the univariate ALT model without predictor variables (Wan, 2002; Bollen and Curran, 2004). The loadings for the QI intercept factor (e.g., the initial status) are all fixed to 1.0, indicating that this factor has a fixed and equal influence on the QI variable. Because the quality changes of individual nursing facilities are least likely to be linear, the loadings for the slope factor (the growth trend) are not completely fixed at the known values of the time measure (in this case, the year indicators 1, 2, 3, 4, 5, and 6 for 1998–2003). The time scores for 1997 (the first year of study) and 2003 (the last year of study) are fixed at 0 and 6 while the remaining time scores are free-estimated in between. Because we are primarily interested in understanding relationships and individual differences starting from the beginning of the assessed growth process, we place the origin of the time at the initial assessment (Biesanz et al., 2004). This pattern of loadings implies that the slope factor has an increasing but nonlinear growth on the successive measures of a nursing home's QI variable (the rate of reduction in incidents of pressure ulcers, physical restraint use, and catheter use). The correlation between intercept and slope are also included in the model to examine whether facilities with high initial quality scores improve at a higher rate (Ferrer, Hamagami, and McArdle, 2004). However, this approach yields poor goodness-of-fit statistics.

The autoregressive latent trajectory (growth curve) model can be extended to include time-constant and time-varying predictor variables, so that the net influence of one causal variable on an endogenous QI variable can be determined. Using ALT modeling, this chapter examines whether or not nursing homes' rehabilitative service use, nurse staffing, and nursing care adequacy, as time-specific exogenous variables, improve the quality of resident care when the effects of facility and market characteristics (contextual variables) are simultaneously considered. The ALT model will also produce factor loadings that show the net effect of nurse staffing, nursing care adequacy, and rehabilitation services on QI for each wave.

In performing the longitudinal analysis, we use Mplus, a statistical modeling program that provides researchers with a flexible multivariate analysis tool to analyze both categorical and continuous variables (L. Muthén and B. Muthén, 1998). In this analysis, only statistically significant results ($p < 0.05$) are discussed. The goodness of fit of the growth curve model is determined by statistics such as chi-square, p-value, comparative fit index (CFI), Tucker-Lewis Index (TLI), root mean square error approximation (RMSEA), and standardized root mean square error (SRMSE).

Findings

Descriptive Analysis

Summary descriptive statistics are shown in table 5.1. The mean nursing care deficiency score ranges from 0.547 to 0.649 across 7 years. The maximum score over the 7 years is 8. The mean QI shows a decline in poor resident outcomes from 1997 to 2003. The scores are -10.527 in 1997 and -8.454 in 2003, respectively. The rate of using rehabilitative service varies across nursing homes. Some facilities provide none of these services, while others provide them to all residents. Nursing staffing decreases slightly over the 7 years, from 4.523 to 3.550 hours per resident day, with great variation from facility to facility. It is important to note that no apparent changes were observed for nurse staffing and rehabilitation when growth curve modeling was performed for each of these exogenous variables.

The average nursing home in 1997 had 118 beds, 14.7 percent Medicare recipients, and an average acuity index of 10.202. In 1997, there was on average 5.4 percent of people aged 75 or older in the United States. In 1997, the percentages of nursing homes that were identified as for-profit, chain members, urban and South-based were 65.97, 56.78, 69.97, and 8.03 percent, respectively.

Table 5.1 Summary Descriptive Statistics, 1997–2003
(N = 11,197)

Variable name	Mean	Standard deviation
NCD97	0.608	0.987
NCD98	0.583	0.959
NCD99	0.581	0.955
NCD00	0.625	0.983
NCD01	0.649	0.975
NCD02	0.604	0.969
NCD03	0.547	0.909
QI97	−10.527	14.055
QI98	−9.755	12.194
QI99	−9.241	11.487
QI00	−8.720	10.709
QI01	−8.586	10.612
QI02	−8.772	9.560
QI03	−8.454	8.998
Reh97	.199	17.074
Reh98	.195	15.848
Reh99	.172	14.898
Reh00	.171	14.144
Reh01	.182	14.161
Reh02	.192	13.989
Reh03	.205	14.673
NS97	4.523	23.892
NS98	4.214	23.150
NS99	4.218	18.328
NS00	4.217	13.965
NS01	4.063	15.858
NS02	3.618	3.992
NS03	3.550	3.956
Bed size	118.125	78.799
% Elders 75+	5.40	2.20
Average acuity	10.202	1.640
% Medicare	14.70	22.50

	Percentage
For-profit facilities	65.97
Chain affiliation	56.78
Urban	69.97
South	8.03

Note: NCD = nursing care deficiency citations; NS = nurse staffing index; Reh = rate of use of rehabilitative services.

The Measurement Model of Quality Index

A single-indicator growth curve model of nursing homes' resident outcomes was performed for the quality index (QI) repeated measures (1997–2003), using ALT modeling. This initial model has a chi-square value of 69.058 with 8 degrees of freedom. The root mean squared error of approximation (RMSEA = 0.026) shows an excellent fit of the model. The linear growth variances for both intercept and slope are statistically significant. The correlation between the intercept and the slope is -0.868 with a critical value of -6.750 (statistically significant). The facilities with lower QI for the earlier years had improved resident outcomes in the later years. Autoregression coefficients of QI measures (with statistically significant standardized coefficients of $-0.075, 0.139, 0.161, 0.185, 0.250,$ and 0.209 for the period of 1997–2003, respectively) reveal that the prior QI value did positively influence the latter value in the six intervals of QI measurement. Finally, the six quality indexes (QI_98 to QI03), with R^2 values of 0.723 in 1998, 0.480 in 1999, 0.487 in 2000, 0.460 in 2001, 0.572 in 2002, and 0.585 in 2003, show statistically significant associations with the change trajectories of the QI measurement.

Cross-Lagged Models of Improvement in Residents' Outcomes

In exploring the one-year lagged effects of nurse staff and rehabilitation variables on resident outcomes without control variables, we formulated and validated a cross-lagged model. Figure 5.1 shows the standardized parameter estimates of the effects. The goodness-of-fit statistics show that this model is poorly fitted with the data, with a chi-square value of 8,883 (166 degrees of freedom and p-value of 0.00), CFI of 0.935, TLI of 0.918, and RMSEA of 0.068. Several findings are noted: (1) the rehabilitation variable was relatively stable over time in comparison with nurse staffing, (2) the nurse staffing variable had no statistically significant lagged effect on resident outcomes, and (3) the lagged effects of rehabilitation variable on resident outcomes were inconsistent. The direct and indirect effects of the adequacy of nursing care and rehabilitation services on resident outcomes of nurse staffing were not statistically significant.

An ALT Model of Quality with Time-Constant and Time-Specific Predictor Variables

By including eight time-invariant predictor variables (contextual and market characteristics) as having direct causal paths with the Time-1 measure (QI_97),

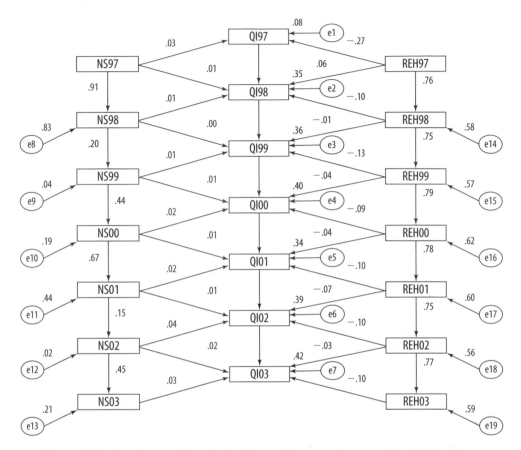

Figure 5.1. A Cross-Lagged Model of the Effects of Nurse Staffing and Rehabilitation on Changes in Resident Outcomes, 1997–2003

intercept (I_qi), and slope (S_qi), we postulated that these variables measured in 1997 directly influenced the change trajectory of each nursing home's QI measure (see figure 5.2). In addition, residual terms were assumed to be correlated, because it was possible that potential predictor variables, such as resident characteristics, had not been included in the prediction.

Table 5.2 shows the results for the ALT model with predictor variables of nursing homes' changes in quality from 1997 to 2003. Eight variables included in the predictive equation of the intercept factor account for 36.2 percent of the variance in I_QI. Six statistically significant predictors of the initial level of QI are: (1) bed size (−.536); (2) for-profit (.056); (3) chain (.021), (4) average

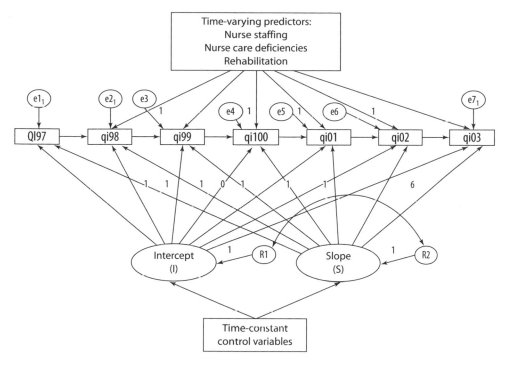

Figure 5.2. An Autoregressive Latent Trajectory Model of the Quality Index in Nursing Homes, with Time-Invariant and Time-Varying Predictors

acuity level (−.073); (5) percent Medicare (0.171); and (6) South (−0.064) and urban (−0.024).

For the slope factor, three of the eight time-constant predictors are statistically significant. The change trajectories in QI are positively associated with bed size (.325), and negatively associated with for-profit (−.082) and percent Medicare (−.139). The eight predictor variables only account for 14.4 percent variation in the slope. The residuals of QI_97 (Time 1), intercept, and slope factors are significantly correlated.

The effects of time-specific predictors (nurse staffing, rehabilitation, and nursing care deficiency citations) on each QI of the 7 years are presented also in Table 5.2. The lagged effect of the prior QI on the latter QI measure is statistically significant for the last 5 years, ranging from 0.223 in 1999 to 0.276 in 2003. Nurse staffing has a positive impact on quality of care, but its impact is negligible in 1999–2003, when the lagged effect of the prior QI measure and the effects of rehabilitation services and nursing care adequacy are simultaneously

Table 5.2 An Autoregressive Latent Trajectory Model for Quality Change, with Time-Invariant and Time-Specific Predictors, 1997–2003

	B	SE	Critical value	b
Intercept (I qi) on time-invariant predictors:				
(R² = .362)				
Bed size	−.704	.014	−48.938	−.536*
For-profit	1.221	.229	5.329	.056*
Chain	.226	.115	1.958	.021*
Average acuity	−.462	.064	−7.187	−.073*
% Medicare	7.854	.657	11.949	.171*
South	−2.435	.385	−6.326	−.064*
Urban	−0.539	.234	−2.308	−.024*
% Elders (75+)	.000	.000	−0.168	−.002
Slope (S qi) on Time-Invariant Predictors:				
(R² = .144)				
Bed size	.055	.003	20.697	.325*
For-profit	−.227	.040	−5.690	−.082*
Chain	−.028	.020	−1.394	−.020
Average acuity	.004	.011	.332	.005
% Medicare	−.823	.120	−6.885	−.139*
South	.123	.067	1.838	.025
Urban	.019	.041	.473	.007
% Elders (75+)	.000	.000	.036	.001
Each period rate on time-specific predictors:				
QI97 on (R² = .547)				
Reh97	.588	.666	.882	.009
NS97	.011	.005	2.304	.018*
NCD97	−.737	.109	−6.794	−.052*
QI98 on (R² = .560)				
QI97	.063	.036	1.743	.072
Reh98	.970	.508	1.910	.017
NS98	.009	.004	2.364	.018*
NCD98	−.498	.009	−5.546	−.039*
QI99 on (R² = .482)				
QI98	.210	.015	14.027	.223*
Reh99	1.297	.398	3.262	.024*
NS99	.004	.004	.994	.007
NCD99	−.200	.081	−2.469	−.017*
QI00 on (R² = .517)				
QI99	.286	.009	31.918	.308*
Reh00	2.203	.381	5.789	.042*
NS00	.007	.005	1.288	.009
NCD00	−.216	.070	−3.073	−.020*

Table 5.2 *Continued*

	B	SE	Critical value	b
QI01 on (R² = .460)				
QI00	.250	.009	27.134	.253*
Reh01	1.567	.386	4.058	.030*
NS01	.003	.005	.536	.004
NCD01	−.353	.074	−4.781	−.033*
QI02 on (R² = .539)				
QI01	.255	.008	30.184	.282*
Reh02	.869	.369	2.354	.018*
NS02	−.004	.016	−.233	−.002
NCD02	−.355	.065	−5.484	−.036*
QI03 on (R² = .561)				
QI02	.263	.010	25.652	.276*
Reh03	.848	.354	2.396	.019
NS03	.020	.015	1.268	.009
NCD03	−.211	.066	−3.216	−.021*

Note: B = unstandardized parameter estimate; SE = standard error; b = standardized parameter estimate; and critical value = a test of the statistical significance of B. NCD = nursing care deficiency citations; NS = nurse staffing index; Reh = rate of use of rehabilitation services; QI = a weighted index of
improved resident outcomes.
    *Statistically significant at $p \leq 0.05$; Goodness-of-fit (GOF) statistics: chi-square = 345.575 with 178
degrees of freedom; Comparative fit index (CFI) = .996; Tucker-Lewis Index (TLI) = .995; Root mean
square error of approximation (RMSEA) = .009.

considered. The rate of rehabilitative service use is positively associated with
the QI of resident outcomes in 4 (1999–2002) of the 6 years. The autoregressive
latent trajectory model with predictor variables shows an excellent fit to the
data, with a chi-square value of 345.575 (178 degrees of freedom), CFI of 0.996,
TLI of 0.995, and RMSEA of 0.009.

Conclusion

The SPO framework is a theoretically informed approach to a longitudinal study
of nursing home quality (Wan, 2003; Unruh and Wan, 2004; Mor, 2005; Goodson, Jang, and Rantz, 2008). Autoregressive latent trajectory modeling is a powerful analytical tool for investigating net effects of nursing-related factors on
the improvement of resident outcomes in nursing homes, when contextual
and lagged variables are simultaneously considered. Nursing systems research

substantially benefits from longitudinal analysis of outcome variables at the facility level.

In the analysis of QI, the intercept factor was well predicted by six contextual and facility characteristics variables, accounting for 36.2 percent of the variance. Bed size was the strongest predictor, while the percentage of people over 75 in the county and urban location was not statistically significant. The slope factor or change trajectory was only weakly predicted by eight time-constant predictors, accounting for 14.4 percent of the variance. It is interesting to note that the higher rate of changes in QI was observed in facilities having large bed size, being not for-profit, having residents with lower average acuity levels, and caring for fewer Medicare recipients.

The autoregressive part of the analysis of QI measures shows that controlling for the lagged effect of the prior QI measure—rehabilitative service use—had a positive, significant influence on the change trajectories from 1999 to 2002; however, no influence was observed in the earlier years. Nurse staffing did not exert much influence on the change trajectories, except in 1997 and 1998, when the influences of other factors were simultaneously considered in the analysis. In addition, results show that there is a significant negative relationship between QI measures and nursing care adequacy, but the relationships between nurse staffing, rehabilitative service, and nursing care adequacy were inconsistent.

The combination of the autoregressive model and latent trajectory model in this analysis generates complex results that have partially supported the major hypothesis: nursing homes with higher nurse staffing, more rehabilitative care, and fewer nursing care deficiencies will show improved resident outcomes while controlling for facility characteristics, contextual factors, and lagged effect. The present longitudinal analysis did not include any cross-lagged effects of nursing related variables on QI because the preliminary study shows that nurse staffing does not have lagged impact on QI while rehabilitative care has inconsistent lagged impact on QI. These variables were not strongly associated with each other or with the outcome variable. The analysis also did not consider nursing care deficiencies to be endogenously related to nurse staffing and rehabilitation services.

Future studies should expand the growth curve model with mixture variables by stratifying the total number of nursing homes into relatively homogenous groups. Alternatively, future studies could use an autoregressive parallel growth curve model with nursing care deficiencies as endogenous. Thus the quality of nursing care and resident outcomes can be better investigated in different clusters of facilities with varying system characteristics such as for-profit versus nonprofit nursing homes, South versus non-South region, and small- versus large-sized homes, and low versus high concentration of residents with Medicare for nursing home care. Additional time-varying predictor variables, including physical and cognitive functional status and other case mix measures, should also be identified from the MDS database to study the improvement of resident outcomes. Further, the relationship between specific clinic factors and the quality of life of residents should be explored (Degenholtz et al., 2008; Alexander and Hearld, 2009). A systematic assessment of the relationship between nursing home productivity/efficiency and quality of care should be investigated. Those steps can generate new knowledge to guide the systems reform toward more effective as well as efficient management practices in nursing home care.

CHAPTER 6

Policies regarding Minimum Staffing Levels

The quality of care in nursing homes continues to be problematic (U.S. Department of Health and Human Services, 1999; Breen and Zhang, 2008). A well-motivated, skilled, and appropriately deployed workforce is crucial to the success of care system delivery and to reach the quality standards of care (Prins and Henderickx, 2007). There is a general belief that nurse staffing has decreased in nursing homes over the years. However, a systematic analysis of the trends and patterns of nurse staffing, based on Online Survey Certification and Reporting (OSCAR) data from 1997 to 2007, shows a different picture. Controlling for facility size and ownership, Seblega et al. (2009) reported that more nursing homes increased—rather than decreased—licensed practical nurse (LPN) and nursing assistant (NA) hours per resident day between 1997 and 2007. On the other hand, more nursing homes decreased—rather than increased—registered nurse (RN) hours per resident day and skill mix during the same time period.

Two major concerns are the quality of nursing care and the adequacy of nurse staffing, believed to be a contributor to the quality of nursing care (Harrington et al., 2000a, 2000b). Few studies have attempted to ascertain the actual minimum levels of nursing staff needed in nursing homes (Unruh and Wan, 2004; Zhang et al., 2006; Zhang and Wan, 2007; Breen, Matusitz, and Wan, 2009). Of those that have, minimum staffing is considered to be a measure below which quality is acceptable, but above which quality continues to improve at the same rate with additional staffing. Such an approach to minimum nurse staffing looks at the staffing/quality relationship in absolute terms. It does not apply efficiency considerations to additional staffing (Newcomer et al., 2001).

There is a direct effect of the RN-to-total nurse staffing ratio on serious deficiencies in nursing homes (Kim, Harrington, and Greene, 2009). To date, the federal Nursing Home Reform Act (NHRA), as part of the Omnibus Budget Reconciliation Act (OBRA) of 1987, requires minimum staffing levels for registered nurses (RNs) and licensed practical nurses (LPNs), and minimum educational training for nursing assistants [(NAs) Omnibus Budget Reconciliation Act, 1987]. The NHRA requires Medicare- and Medicaid-certified nursing homes to have: (1) an RN director of nursing (DON); (2) an RN on duty at least 8 hours per day, 7 days a week; (3) a licensed nurse (RN or LPN) on duty the remainder of the time; and (4) a minimum of 75 hours of training for nurse aides. Legal mandates and policy allow the DONs to also serve in the capacity as the RN on duty in facilities with fewer than 60 residents. In addition, NHRA requires nursing homes to supply adequate staff and services to attain or maintain the highest possible level of physical, mental, and psychosocial well-being of each resident (Omnibus Budget Reconciliation Act, 1987; Harrington, 2001a). Total licensed nursing requirements converted to hours per resident day (HPRD) in a facility with 100 residents are about 0.30 HPRD (Harrington and Millman, 2001), or 30 hours per day. Despite setting a precedent, this requirement does not provide specific nurse-to-resident staffing ratios for RNs, LPNs, or NAs, nor does it require any minimum level of staffing for NAs whatsoever.

The NHRA also designed and established "Residents' Bill of Rights" for nursing home residents. These rights were implemented across nursing homes in the United States to ensure that adequate care and dignified respect were being delivered to residents in institutionalized care settings. The rights, according to the NHRA, are as follows:

- The right to freedom from abuse, mistreatment, and neglect
- The right to freedom from physical restraints
- The right to privacy
- The right to accommodation of medical, physical, psychological, and social needs
- The right to participate in resident and family groups
- The right to be treated with dignity
- The right to exercise self-determination
- The right to communicate freely
- The right to participate in the review of one's care plan and to be fully informed in advance about any changes in care, treatment, or change of status in the facility
- The right to voice grievances without discrimination or reprisal.

Other than the instructions to provide "sufficient" staff, the fact that a facility of 50 residents has basically the same staffing requirements as a facility of 200 indicates the lack of specificity and adequacy of these federal requirements (Zhang et al., 2006). Most states have additional requirements above and beyond the federal mandates. In one study, 15 states had higher RN standards and 25 states had higher licensed nursing standards than the federal minimum staffing requirements. Eight states required an RN on duty 24 hours per day for facilities with 100 or more residents. Thirty-three states required minimum staffing for nursing assistants (Harrington and Millman, 2001). The highest overall staffing requirement is in California: 3.2 hours per resident day, excluding administrative nurses (Harrington, 2001b).

The federal government as well as researchers recognize the importance of further addressing nurse staffing standards, and some studies have explored specific thresholds. Harrington et al. (2000a, 2000b) provided recommendations on minimum standards for nurse staffing levels based on the expertise of a focus group of national experts on staffing and quality in nursing homes. The expert panel recommended one full-time RN director of nursing and one RN supervisor on duty at all times (24 hours per day, 7 days per week) in all nursing homes across the country. In facilities with 100 or more beds, the same panel recommended a full-time RN assistant director of nursing and a full-time RN director of in-service education. In facilities with fewer than 100 beds, these positions should be proportionally adjusted for size. RN hours per resident day should total 1.15. Recommendations for LPNs were 0.70 hours per resident day, whereas NAs were suggested at 2.70 hours per resident day. Total nursing staff hours were recommended to be at least 4.55 per resident day. These ratios were higher than the actual average ratios reported in the OSCAR data. While this study was instructive in listing specific minimum ratios for each type of nursing staff member, the staffing ratios established qualitatively by experts would gain credence if bolstered by a quantitative analysis led by statistical and health care experts (Zhang et al., 2006; Zhang and Wan, 2007).

In 2000 and 2001, the CMS and Abt Associates, Inc., published two consecutive reports quantitatively analyzing the appropriateness of minimum nurse staffing ratios in nursing homes (see Zhang et al., 2006). In phase II of their studies, the organizations reported the identification of a point at which no further benefits could be obtained by increasing the nursing staff (Kramer and Fish, 2001; Zhang et al., 2006). For RNs, this point was 0.75 hours per resident day for the long-term care measures; for licensed staff members (RNs and LPNs), it was 1.3 hours, and for NAs, 2.8 hours. However, these thresholds for different nursing staff represent maximums, that is, the question of how far below this threshold the facility could be staffed before quality was seriously undermined and could not be ascertained.

Interestingly, the calculation of thresholds was based on only the worst 10 percent of nursing homes in terms of quality of care. No information is available for quality thresholds above the tenth percentile. In addition, the odds ratio was used to judge the nurse staffing threshold, but the relationship between staffing and quality is uniform throughout the logistic model. Finally, the study sample was from a limited number of states (Zhang et al., 2006), thus jeopardizing the validity of the study.

Hendrix and Foreman (2001) examined optimal staffing levels from the vantage point of minimizing the costs of decubitus ulcers (pressure sores). While Hendrix and Foreman identified cost levels for RNs and NAs that minimized the costs of decubitus ulcers (they did not find an optimal point for LPNs), they did not constrain their analysis to any given level of incidence of decubitus ulcers. Hence, the optimal staffing levels ascertained in this study were those that minimized costs, but at an unknown and not necessarily optimal level of quality of care (Zhang et al., 2006).

The positive relationship between nurse staffing levels and the quality of nursing home care has been widely demonstrated (Newcomer et al., 2001; Wan, 2003; Unruh and Wan, 2004; Scott-Cawiezell et al., 2007). However, Castle and Engberg (2008) noted that staffing size may be a necessary but not sufficient means for achieving high quality of nursing home care. The professional staff mix, stability and use of agency staff should be considered when nurse staffing is being examined. Studies have associated more RN or licensed nurses hours per resident day with better care, fewer deficiency citations, a higher probability of discharge, a lower probability of death, fewer pressure ulcers, better mental and functional status of residents, and less use of restraints (Wan, Zhang, and Unruh, 2006). Furthermore, nursing homes receive federal audit deficiency citations if they are found to be using restraints inappropriately (Hillmer et al., 2005).

State survey reports as well as research have started to underscore the reality that inadequate nursing care processes lead to poor resident outcomes. Failure to provide comprehensive care plans for residents and poor resident assessment are among the top 10 deficiencies cited by state surveyors (Wan, Zhang, and Unruh, 2006). Braun (1991) found that nursing processes such as positioning, catheter care, and personal hygiene lower mortality and increase the likelihood of discharge among VA nursing home residents. Another study found that facilities with more catheter use, less skin care, and low resident participation in organized activities tended to have negative resident outcomes (Spector and Takada, 1991).

This chapter discussed the policies and regulations regarding the minimum nursing home medical practitioner levels/numbers/ratios within the nursing home care facility context. It is crucial to recognize the Nursing Home Reform Act, as well as stipulations required by the CMS, strongly recommend and attempt to enforce that certain numbers of registered nurses, nursing assistants, and other health practitioners in the nursing home setting are secured and employed at all times. Such staffing levels optimize the chances of sufficient care delivery to the nursing home residents, that is, those who are cared for directly by the practitioners with whom they trust and receive treatment. Furthermore, the staffing adequacy coupled with continuing education (Mezey, Mitty, and Burger, 2008), training (Wiener et al., 2009), and certification (Squillace et al., 2009) could ensure better quality of care delivered in nursing homes. The next chapter takes an economic viewpoint to assess nursing home efficiency and its connection to the quality of care in nursing homes. The roles of market competition and payer mix are also examined.

CHAPTER 7

The Relationship between Efficiency and the Quality of Care

When considering how market competition, staffing issues, and payer mix distributions affect the stability and economic status of nursing homes, one must understand an economic view of efficiency and its complex connection to the quality of care delivered in nursing homes.

Assessing Efficiency

Economists define three main types of efficiency: (1) technical, (2) allocative, and (3) productive (Zhang, Unruh, and Wan, 2008). Technical efficiency is the maximum possible output from a given set of inputs. Allocative efficiency is the most efficient combination of inputs, given their prices and production technology. Productive or total economic efficiency is when both technological and allocative efficiency exist. In addition, economists also speak of X-efficiency, which is the maximum effective use of inputs under internal motivational and external environmental and market pressures. X-efficiency differs from technical efficiency in that technical efficiency assumes that profit-maximizing behavior in a market environment motivates the efficient use of given inputs to produce the maximum outputs, whereas X-efficiency assumes that other internal behaviors and external situations may motivate inefficient use of inputs (Zhang, Unruh, and Wan, 2008). For managerial and environmental reasons, in actuality, organizations may not minimize costs and maximize profits. X-inefficiency is the degree of difference between the maximal possible effectiveness of the use of inputs and the actual effectiveness (Anderson et al., 2005).

X-efficiency applies to this analysis because the profit motive is less strong in nursing homes than in non-health care markets and market mechanisms also are weaker. The environmental pressure exerted or produced by the Medicare prospective payment system represents a coercive nonmarket mechanism (Zhang, Unruh, and Wan, 2008). Managers may not have the knowledge, resources, or motivation to find new efficiencies in light of reimbursement cuts. Attempts to reduce input costs to levels that match the lower revenues may drive the use of inputs below what is needed to maintain the same level and quality of outputs (Zhang, Unruh, and Wan, 2008).

Reductions in public reimbursement are intended to save or preserve public resources while encouraging efficiency, yet they may have unintended corollaries. If facilities have already achieved a high level of efficiency, or if not enough resources are available to move to a more efficient level, the cuts in reimbursement may lead those facilities to reduce essential inputs—such as nursing staff—who are indispensable to maintain the necessary and acceptable level of quality of care (Unruh, Zhang, and Wan, 2006). While prospective payment systems are the most efficient payment systems (Zinn et al., 2003), fixed reimbursements must be carefully developed from ongoing evidence-based research; they must be adjusted for the case-mix or acuity (Feng et al., 2006).

Plagued by continuing problems related to quality of care and operating under a fixed payment system, the nursing home industry believes that a policy of pay-for-performance might encourage or more substantially boost both quality and efficiency. A financial incentive could be provided in advance of efficiency-enhancing changes (such as physical or work redesign) to affect changes leading to higher efficiency. Quality will be encouraged and reinforced when facilities meet their quality indicators (Unruh, Zhang, and Wan, 2006; Zhang and Wan, 2007).

According to Zhang, Unruh, and Wan (2008), recent changes in reimbursement policy have had a significant negative impact on efficiency. Higher nurse staffing contributes to lower efficiency only when efficiency is not adjusted for quality of care. Various organizational and market factors also play significant roles in all efficiency models.

Nurse staffing levels and skill mix may also influence efficiency (Zhang, Unruh, and Wan, 2008). In general, the more staff members employed for any unit of output, the lower the efficiency. Nonetheless, this particular relationship may not be linear; at some point, fewer staff members may lead to disorganized care and poorer resident outcomes—lower output—(Zhang et al., 2006). Because the skilled nursing homes in the United States are about 66 percent for-profit, the issue of ownership is important. It is believed that the incentive for efficiency is reduced in nonprofit facilities as they have more stakeholders, have more varied goals, and may receive charitable subsidies (Zhang, Unruh, and Wan, 2008). Empirical studies generally indicate that for-profit status has a positive effect on efficiency (Knox, Blankmeyer, and Stutzman, 2001). A higher occupancy rate may indicate the efficient use of inputs or it may be related to losses in efficiency because of congestion or overpopulation.

Ozcan, Wogen, and Mau (1998), however, found that occupancy rate is positively associated with efficiency. Economies of scale—when costs increase by a lesser amount than when output increases—is another factor that affects efficiency in nursing homes. Larger facilities and members of chains may have economies of scale because they can share technology and resources and may have bargaining power (Zhang, Unruh, and Wan, 2008). Anderson, Lewis, and Webb (1999) found less cost efficiency in nursing homes that are members of chains. To the contrary, when costs and profits are analyzed, nursing homes in chains are found to be more efficient (Knox, Blankmeyer, and Stutzman, 2001).

Market competition may affect efficiency by motivating an organization to produce efficiently to compete successfully. The Herfindahl-Hirschman Index indicates the number of firms in the market. Higher values indicate fewer firms in the market. Studies applying the Herfindahl-Hirschman Index have found that market competition increases efficiency (Zhang, Unruh, and Wan, 2008). Payer mix may affect efficiency if nursing homes with a high concentration of low reimbursement payers may be motivated to be more efficient. For example, most studies demonstrate that a high proportion of Medicaid recipients is a predictor or strong indicator of efficiency (Ozcan, Wogen, and Mau, 1998; Grabowski, Angelelli, and Mor, 2004).

According to Zhang, Unruh, and Wan (2008), a higher RN-to-resident (registered nurse-to-resident) day ratio and RN nursing staff proportion were found to be related to lower efficiency when efficiency is not adjusted for the quality of care. This situation is to be expected as higher numbers of RNs or skill mix reduces the output-to-input ratio if quality is not considered. However, when efficiency is adjusted for quality, better staffing is associated with improved efficiency (Konetzka, Stearns, and Park, 2008). The probable reason for this link is that reducing RN staff to improve efficiency may compromise quality. Instead, to accomplish efficiency while maintaining quality, the opposite is the case: more RN staffing may be needed. Further, Medicaid rates and revenues have a strong influence on efficiency (Zhang, Unruh, and Wan, 2008).

The Structural Relationship between Efficiency and the Quality of Care

Previous chapters discussed the structure-process-outcome (SPO) aspects of the quality of care in nursing homes. Similarly, we can examine the aspects of cost efficiency, process efficiency, and productive efficiency that comprise the efficiency of nursing home care. Such triadic conceptualizations of efficiency and of the quality of care can guide the development of measurement models, using both cross-sectional and longitudinal data of both domains of nursing home performance.

The Efficiency of Nursing Homes

Figure 7.1 offers a measurement model of nursing home efficiency that reflects cost efficiency, process efficiency, and productive efficiency. The premise for this model is that those three domains of efficiency are not independent. Rather, an oblique relationship among the three domains is expected. Multiple indicators for each aspect of efficiency are used as the output variables; the input variables are the expenses for general services, routine services, and ancillary services. An efficiency score is computed by applying Data Envelopment Analysis (DEA). Originally devised by Charnes, Cooper, and Rhodes (1978), DEA is a quantitative method that computes efficiency scores for decision-making units (DMUs) in comparison to their peer units. DEA has been applied to a variety of research: the assessment of hospital efficiency (Ozcan, Luke, and Haksever, 1992), medical practitioners' efficiency (Ozcan, Jiang, and Pai, 2000), efficiency ratings among organizations dedicated to preserving health care (Rosenman, Siddharthan, and Ahern, 1997), as well as in other health-related contexts (see Ozgen and Ozcan, 2004).

Ozcan, Wogen, and Mau (1998) used DEA to assess the technical efficiency of 324 skilled nursing facilities (SNFs), comparing them by ownership and size. The input variables were the number of beds, participating FTEs, and operational expenses. The output variables were the sum of total inpatient days of Medicare and Medicaid and total private-pay inpatient days. The authors found that for-profit facilities were more efficient than nonprofit facilities. Those with higher percentages of residents receiving Medicare were technically less efficient; however, those with higher percentages of Medicaid recipients and with

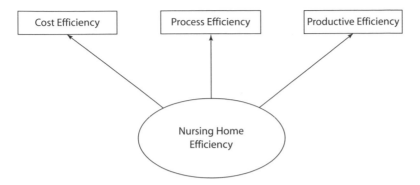

Figure 7.1. The Measurement Model of Efficiency in Nursing Homes

higher occupancy rates were more technically efficient. The medium-sized facilities were more efficient than large or small ones.

According to Nayar and Ozcan (2008, p. 193), DEA is a "useful technique
to assess organizational performance in terms of technical and allocative efficiency." Besides an overview of the reliability and validity of this instrument in
practice, it is important to recognize the specific indicators for measuring each
domain of efficiency. Those are identified as follows: (1) cost efficiency—the
average operating cost per resident is a negative aspect of efficiency, so this inef-
ficiency indicator is inverted: 1/(average operating cost per resident); (2) process efficiency—the average occupancy rate; and (3) productive efficiency —the
three indicators used measure the total skilled nursing inpatient days, the intermediate nursing inpatient days, and other long-term care inpatient days. Figure 7.1 displays this measurement model of efficiency in nursing homes.

Because the efficiency score generated from DEA is constrained within the
unitary boundary, the following calculation is taken: the higher the score observed for a facility, the higher its efficiency level. An aggregated efficiency score
is computed for each facility. Each facility's efficiency level thus can be used to
rank the relative performance of the investigated nursing homes. Using Florida
nursing homes (n = 396) as an example, we computed the DEA score (technical
efficiency) for each facility.

The Quality of Care in Nursing Homes

It is also important to examine the quality of care of nursing home care within
this context. Figure 7.2 presents a measurement model of the quality of nursing

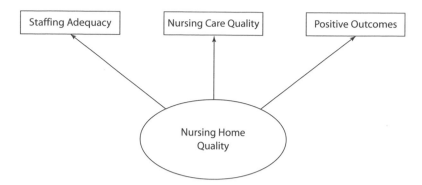

Figure 7.2. The Measurement Model of the Quality of Care in Nursing Homes

home care, reflecting three domains of quality of care: (1) adequacy of staffing; (2) adequacy of nursing care; and (3) residents' outcomes. The indicators measuring each domain are presented below and clarified in the paragraphs that follow.

The number of deficiency citations for staff inadequacy reflects a poor structural aspect of a given nursing home's care. Therefore, this indicator is inverted: 1/(deficiency citations for staffing).

The quality of the actual care is obviously also part and parcel of this discussion. The number of citations for deficiencies in nursing care reflects a poor process aspect of the nursing home's quality of care. This indicator is also inverted: 1/(deficiency citations for quality of nursing care).

According to Wan, Zhang, and Unruh (2006), resident outcomes include the incidence rates for pressure ulcers, for urinary tract infections, and for physical restraints, which are poor resident outcomes. Note that these indicators are inverted to reflect the positive aspects of resident outcomes. Three basic measures are presented: (1) 1/(rate of pressure ulcers); (2) 1/(rate of urinary tract infections); and (3) 1/(rate of physical restraints).

When the quality of care in nursing homes is assessed in terms of its efficiency, note that the quality indicators are treated as the output variables. The input variables are the expenses for general services, routine services, and ancillary services. DEA is applied to arrive at a quality efficiency score. Because the quality efficiency score is also constrained within the unitary boundary, the higher the DEA score, the higher the quality efficiency. The rankings of the 396 nursing homes studied have been computed.

The Relationship between Efficiency and Quality in Nursing Homes

Often there is a trade-off relationship between technical efficiency and quality in the manufacturing industry. However, prominent studies and literature reviews in the health services field show that there is a positive relationship between technical efficiency and the quality of hospital care (Lee and Wan, 2002; Wan, 2002; Nayar and Ozcan, 2008). The relationship between technical efficiency and quality efficiency in nursing homes has not been thoroughly investigated. We postulate that for nursing home care, there is a concurrent effect of technical efficiency on quality efficiency. In addition, we postulate that cross-lagged effects of technical efficiency (TE) and quality efficiency (QE) exist; for example, (1) TE at time 1 affects QE at time 2; and (2) QE at time 1 affects TE at time 2.

The availability of panel data from nursing homes enables us to empirically validate this assumption. First, we examined correlation analysis of the technical efficiency and quality scores of 396 Florida nursing homes for each study year in the cross-sectional analysis. Table 7.1 summarizes the results and delineates a positive relationship between these two dimensions of nursing home performance.

Second, we constructed and validated the cross-lagged effect model, applying longitudinal data with five waves (1999–2003) of the assessment. Figure 7.3 presents the structural relationship between technical efficiency and quality efficiency, assuming that the earlier measure of technical efficiency affects the latter measure of quality (the lagged effect), and that the earlier measure of quality affects the latter measure of the technical effect (the lagged effect). Moreover, better technical efficiency is concurrently associated with higher quality efficiency in nursing home care (concomitant effect). It is interesting to note that technical efficiency scores are highly stable over time, ranging from

Table 7.1 The Correlation between Technical and Quality Efficiency Scores, 1999–2003

	1999	2000	2001	2002	2003
Correlation coefficient	.128*	.343*	.272*	.210*	.088
Significance level	.011	.000	.000	.000	.079

*Statistically significant at $p \leq 0.05$.

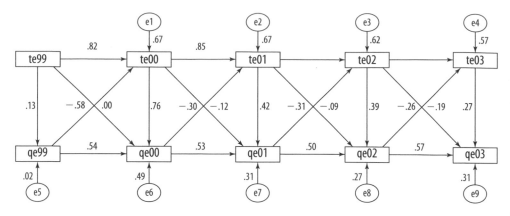

Figure 7.3. The Structural Relationship between Technical Efficiency (TE) and Quality Efficiency (QE) in 396 Florida Nursing Homes: A Cross-Lagged Model without Correlated Residual Errors (e)

0.77 to 0.85. However, quality efficiency scores are moderately stable, ranging from 0.50 to 0.57. This analysis also reveals that a positive and statistically significant effect of technical efficiency on quality efficiency exists: standardized regression coefficients are 0.13, 0.76, 0.42, 0.39, and 0.27, for the years between 1999 and 2003, respectively. This supports the concomitant change of the two performance indicators in nursing homes on the basis of a cross-sectional view of the data. Moreover, the lagged effect of technical efficiency on quality efficiency appears to be negative. This negative effect was much stronger in 1999 (−0.58) but gradually attenuated in later years, with coefficients ranging from −0.30 in 2000 to −0.26 in 2003. Similarly, the lagged effect of quality efficiency on technical efficiency is also negative, but much smaller than that of technical efficiency on quality efficiency: (1) QE99 has no effect on TE00; (2) QE00 has a negative effect on TE01 (−0.12); (3) QE01 has a negative effect on TE02 (−0.09); and (4) QE02 has a negative effect on TE03 (−0.13). Figure 7.3 illustrates these details.

Conclusion

This chapter has analyzed both cross-sectional and longitudinal data for nursing home performance in two major domains: technical efficiency and quality efficiency. We ranked each nursing home in Florida in terms of its performance as measured by technical efficiency and by quality efficiency. Then we examined the potential trade-off relationship between efficiency and quality by cross-sectional analysis and longitudinal panel analysis.

The major findings suggest that there is a positive, concomitant effect of technical efficiency on the quality efficiency of nursing homes. However, the lagged effect of technical efficiency on quality efficiency is negative. This effect appears to be much stronger in 1999 (during the early Medicare Balanced Budget Act period). The negative influence of technical efficiency is gradually attenuated in later years (post-Balanced Budget Act). It is highly possible that nursing homes strove to maximize their productivity under the regulatory and budgetary restraints in the early phase of the Balanced Budget Act period. Such nursing homes have eventually achieved significant improvement in technical efficiency through a learning curve. This minor trade-off relationship between technical efficiency and quality may be dissipated in the future under the Centers for Medicare and Medicaid Services' pay-for-performance initiative. Inspection of the cross-lagged model for the effect of the prior level of quality efficiency on the latter level of technical efficiency level shows a negative relationship, though a weak one. Thus, improving on quality efficiency may not necessarily be detrimental to the technical efficiency of nursing home operation.

It is anticipated that an efficiency equation should include the quality domain. In other words, the improvement of technical efficiency should not be at the expense of the quality of care. An integrated efficiency-quality approach to nursing home care will enable the nursing home sector to be more competitive. Clearly, the objective should be to achieve optimal levels of both efficiency and effectiveness in all respects.

The next chapter discusses how specific information technology services can be helpful in providing additional or supplemental care resources for nursing home practitioners who need increased knowledge to optimally conduct their jobs as caregivers.

Improving Performance and the Quality of Life through Health Informatics

Telemedicine and Ehealth

Information technology (IT) can be tremendously helpful to many industries—to the health care sector—nursing homes, in particular. In addition, decision support technology is especially useful when the services delivered involve medical support and administration to frail and/or elderly individuals. One such practical tool is known as telemedicine, or ehealth. Ehealth is the term for telemedicine that, as Rosen (2000) briefly states, encompasses any database or encyclopedia containing information germane to health, medicine, or pharmacy that is accessible only via the Internet (Breen and Zhang, 2008). Breen and Matusitz (2007) state that ehealth consists of Internet-based services, including sites such as WebMD.com, Medlineplus.gov, Medscape.com, and Mentalhelp.net. WebMD.com (2008), as appropriately listed first above, advertises that its series of subdomains provide the finest quality and quantity of services for medical practitioners and consumers, including a convenient and user-friendly means by which to navigate through the multilevel, multidimensional medical care system. The front page of WebMD.com displays the vast resources this site offers to the medical and public communities. To differentiate telemedicine categorically from ehealth—which represents a subtype of the "telemedicine umbrella" —and to clearly recognize the distinction between these two largely researched topics, one must first comprehensively define telemedicine (Breen and Matusitz, 2007; Matusitz and Breen, 2007; Breen and Zhang, 2008). Telemedicine encompasses telecommunications technologies to aid the delivery and exchange of clinical health care at a distance (Turner, 2003). This delivery method was originally designed to specifically target and benefit patients (Wright, 1998; Wootton, 2001; Breen and Matusitz, 2007; Breen and Zhang, 2008).

When we consider telecommunication technologies that enable communication between medical practitioners and patients, we typically think of familiar or sometimes advanced devices, such as radio, television, telegraphy, telephony, fax machines, interactive television units, and videoconferencing—all of which can be categorized as telemedicine services [(they are telemedicine applications only when applied to serve medical practitioners in health care transactions to patients or consumers at a distance; Conrad, 1998; Matusitz and Breen, 2007; Breen and Zhang, 2008)]. To introduce and promote the employment of ehealth or telemedicine services into nursing home environments, it makes sense to iterate how the devices mentioned earlier, when used in health care functions, performed effectively in facilitating communication between medical providers and their patients (Matusitz and Breen, 2007). A similar degree of satisfaction was observed when these telemedicine applications were used in medically-based settings such as training, research, and administration (Breen and Zhang, 2008).

Because of the distance hurdle that telemedicine and ehealth applications are capable of transcending, Preston, Brown, and Hartley (1992) were convinced from their own research that telemedicine would be especially useful in secluded towns and communities deficient in good-quality health care services —rural areas, mountains, remote islands, and arctic climates. Wright (1998) followed this research and later released publications that telemedicine would be effective in developing and Third World countries. Given the efficacy of telemedicine services, as noted by these scholars in their work in both metropolitan and more rural or remote regions, Breen and Zhang (2008, p. 189) made the argument that ehealth services "would prove valuable when actively used by nursing staff in a variety of nursing homes, regardless of the structure and organization of the nursing home (e.g., nursing home chains in urban and rural areas, for-profit or nonprofit homes, etc)."

Matusitz and Breen (2007) addressed that medical practitioners on their own usually lack the abilities and knowledge to reach the level and quickness of information delivered using ehealth services. In addition, because telemedicine, and especially ehealth services, have shown to reduce many exhausting costs associated with health services in patient care and treatment, Breen and Zhang (2008, p. 189) made the point that "rural and disadvantaged nursing home facilities would benefit tremendously from having a cost-effective method of obtaining health-related information." To bolster their claim, Turner, Thomas, and Reinsch (2004) asserted that ehealth is a more rapid and convenient alternative, as well as a more cost-effective method, for accessing health care information, rather than the traditional and generally costly physical interactions between practitioners and patients in clinical settings. Matusitz and Breen (2007) further contended that ehealth services have the potential to ease several issues that telemedicine has forced itself into the medical system, such as licensing issues, patient privacy, and insurance reimbursement.

A number of publications have documented the quantity and frequency of ehealth service use among practitioners in a variety of specialties and settings: psychiatry, pathology, dermatology, cardiology, in intensive care units, and in emergency rooms where surgery is performed (Turner, 2003; Matusitz and Breen, 2007). According to Breen and Zhang (2008, p. 190), "many of these relate to types of care needed and applied in nursing home settings." In fact, WebMD.com is the preferred source for most medical practitioners (Matusitz and Breen, 2007, 2008). One of the most critical financial benefits revealed within the WebMD.com site for medical practitioners, in particular, is that "its products and services streamline administrative and clinical processes, promote efficiency and reduce costs by facilitating information exchange, and enhance communication and electronic transactions between healthcare participants" (WebMD.com, 2008, p. 5). Even more ambitiously, WebMD.com freely offers "disease and treatment information, pharmacy and drug information, and an array of forums and interactive e-communities where practitioners and consumers can correspond using specialized e-messages" (Breen and Zhang, 2008, p. 190). WebMD.com doesn't cease there in its cost-free provisions to medical practitioners and its potential benefits to nursing home settings, in particular; this site offers to medical practitioners training courses that can eliminate the associated expenses involved in inviting a specialist in the field to lecture in person (WebMD.com, 2008).

In 2005, WebMD.com reported that more than 240 million people visit the site every year. Breen and Zhang (2008) asserted that the rapidly rising use of the Internet, combined with worldwide web surfing for health care information (Rice and Katz, 2001; Breen and Matusitz, 2007; Matusitz and Breen, 2007, 2008), means that medical professionals should embrace and use the Internet in nursing home settings across metropolitan, suburban, and rural sectors. Advancing that argument, Mitka (2003) asserted that ehealth services improved the delivery of psychiatric treatment to residents in rural nursing homes.

Breen and Zhang (2008) proposed theoretical explanations for why ehealth would enhance the quality of care, resident satisfaction, and clinical outcomes

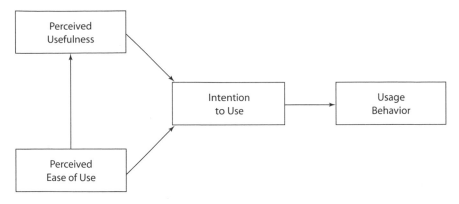

Figure 8.1.The Technology Acceptance Model . *Source*: Davis (1989)

in nursing home settings. The first one they identified is a popular theory commonly referred to as the technology acceptance model [(TAM; Davis, 1989)]. Tersely stated, this model postulates that "the perceived usefulness and ease of use influence and shape a person's willingness and motivation to use a system" (Breen and Zhang, 2008, p. 190). Figure 8.1 illustrates the components of the TAM construct; the model's relevance to the applicability of ehealth services in nursing home care can be seen.

Hu et al., (1999) as well as Breen and Matusitz (2007) contend that many forms of information technology in the medical setting are becoming increasingly welcomed, accepted, and used for diverse health care functions. Because it is well established that technology flows amply throughout the health care industry (Hu et al., 1999; Turner, 2003; Matusitz and Breen, 2007), prompt integration of ehealth into nursing home care is anticipated (Breen and Zhang, 2008).

How can this assertion be put forth that swift adoption of ehealth services will transpire? As Davis (1989) would postulate, ehealth services, within the direct context of nursing home care delivery and quality, would improve employee performance among nursing home staff—reason enough for nursing homes to accept such technology. Further, Matusitz and Breen (2007) assert that the health care industry prefers integrating technology into operations when applications are simple to use. Davis (1989) agrees as he believes that technological systems are more acceptable and adoptable when such services are free of effort and complex involvement.

Another theory asserted by Breen and Zhang (2008) that supports the accep-

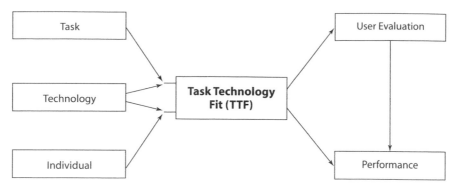

Figure 8.2. The Task Technology Fit Model. *Source*: Goodhue and Thompson (1995)

tance of ehealth in nursing homes is known as the theory of task technology fit (TTF), proposed by Goodhue and Thompson (1995). TTF posits that "IT is more likely to have a positive impact on individual performance and be used if the capabilities of the IT match the tasks that the user must perform" (Goodhue and Thompson, 1995, p. 215). Figure 8.2 illustrates the TTF model and reveals how the contents of this model can relate to the efficacy of such ehealth services in nursing home care.

Ehealth services are intended to supply supplemental knowledge and advice to medical practitioners when they are treating patients. In this case, the patients are nursing home residents. Individual staff performance will be improved because ehealth services, such as WebMD.com, provide direct benefits for the staff members diagnosing and treating residents' health problems. Hu et al. (1999) would agree that these perceived benefits of ehealth in nursing home contexts should grow with regard to physician acceptance. Matusitz and Breen (2008) report similar findings.

When nurses and other medical practitioners who staff nursing homes lack adequate knowledge and skill in physiology and esoteric medical matters, the care they deliver will be inadequate. Integrating ehealth into nursing home care offers a type of encyclopedia that health practitioners in nursing home environments can readily access to obtain the information they need to reach firm decisions when directing care plans and delivery for nursing home residents. Breen and Zhang (2008, p. 191) predict that ehealth services will be "most beneficial within nursing homes that provide specialty care units (i.e., residents with dementia, cancer, cardiovascular problems, and stroke victims), as more complicated and comprehensive care is needed along with vast knowledge in these complex areas of medical care." Breen and Zhang (2008) also point out that, according to the specific attributes of nursing homes and the residents who receive in-patient care at those facilities, underfunded or underprivileged nursing homes would benefit most from using ehealth, that is, computer-based medical databases or online health sites.

In related research described in chapter 4, Zhang et al. (2006, p. 5) examined the "minimum nurse staffing thresholds necessary to achieve both quality and efficiency in nursing homes." They corroborated that the quality in nursing homes demands allocating more financial resources to nurse staffing. In other words, using ehealth services to ameliorate inefficiencies by giving staff greater access to health information via the Internet is sensible. In the same train of thought, smaller-staffed nursing home units that may not be able to allocate more finances toward the hiring of increased nursing staff can use ehealth to their advantage in serving the lower numbers of staff already employed.

The hope is that other countries will be able to adopt these theoretical ideals. Specifically, nursing homes outside of the United States can realize the gravity of deficiencies in U.S. nursing homes—integrating ehealth services into their routine care assessments and delivery may enhance resident care and outcomes. The most fundamental and vital objectives that nursing homes seek to achieve are to provide salubrious, sustaining atmospheres for debilitated or compromised inpatient individuals who require continuous support and medical intervention. Without optimal resources to ensure the most efficacious treatments to nursing home residents—in the United States or elsewhere—attaining the crucial goal of minimizing deficiencies in nursing homes is unlikely.

Another highly relevant resource available on the Internet is known as the Florida Teaching Nursing Home program—a clinical assessment tool that is available by visiting www.geriu.org. This particular program also provides specific information on all kinds of issues, injuries, interventions, and treatments necessary for being an effective caregiver in a nursing home care setting. For instance, educational articles are provided on topics such as pain, falls, depression, and improving the quality of care for nursing home residents. Such a resource can be timely when these kinds of problems occur. Reviewing this material before becoming a nursing home practitioner, as well as refreshing one's knowledge when working in a nursing home care setting, can be beneficial in learning the basics and common occurrences in nursing homes. Besides ehealth services, the Teaching Nursing Home program is another excellent example of an information technology tool that can be used for the direct benefit of nursing home care providers and residents.

Informatics Research in Health and Elder Care

The nursing home industry is a labor-intensive service sector that requires a high-touch and low-tech systems of delivering care. The quality of care in nursing homes cannot be easily optimized without firm knowledge of which practices and techniques work and which do not. Such knowledge stems from scientific information generated from practice-based research, and this research relies on routine data collection and monitoring performance with benchmarked facilities in the same region or state.

Informatics research is a specialty area that integrates health science, computer science, information science, decision science, and management/organizational science to manage and communicate data, information, and knowledge in health care practices and management roles (Wan, 2002; Wan and Lee, 2009). Nursing home informatics, then, facilitates the integration of data, information, and knowledge to support residents, care providers, health care executives, and owners in their decision making in all roles and settings. As Wan (2006) defines nursing home informatics research, it is a systematic process of compiling, analyzing, and simulating data to produce verified and replicated findings from observed facts or phenomena. The endpoint or ultimate outcome expected of this research endeavor is to produce clinical and executive decision support systems that can improve the efficiency and effectiveness of nursing home care practices and the quality of nursing home care management.

Strategies for Informatics Research in Nursing Homes

Informatics research in the nursing home realm is distinct; it requires a clear understanding apart from general informatics research or health care informatics research. According to Wan (2006), the analytical strategies for informatics research in nursing homes are (1) the formulation of a data warehouse for exploration, (2) data mining, (3) the application of confirmatory statistical analysis, (4) simulation via an interface with computer and information system technologies, and (5) translational research. These elements are illustrated in figure 8.3.

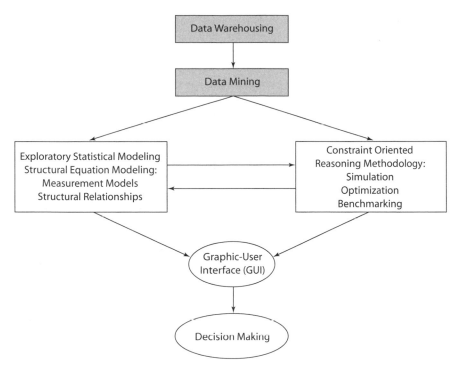

Figure 8.3. Analytical Strategies for Informatics Research in Nursing Homes. *Source*: From "Healthcare informatics research: From data to evidence-based practice" Figure 2 of Wan (2006, p. 5). With kind permission of Springer Science and Business Media

Data Warehousing

Data warehousing is the systematic structuring of data within a theoretically informed framework shared by a disciplinary focus, with the intent to produce useful information for exploration. Analysts extract data from multiple sources (e.g., MDS (Minimum Data Set), OSCAR (Online Survey Certification and Reporting), Medicare, Medicaid, and the Area Resource File (ARF)] to build a relational database. A theoretically specified framework guides data compilation and classifies and populates the study variables uniformly in a logically organized nosological (a branch of medical science that deals with listings or categorizations of diseases) system. A current approach to data structuring is to use data-sharing designs that enable the pooling or pushing of data systems from multiple sources or the units of long-term care institutions. Personal identifiers are encrypted to ensure confidentiality and security of the shared data. At present, the CMS's OSCAR and MDS data systems are not structured as data ware-housing, even though these systems are otherwise feasible for constructing an integrated data structure that researchers and policy analysts would find convenient. The Department of Health and Human Services, under the National Committee on Vital and Health Statistics, should advocate and support the establishment of an integrated data system that could monitor nursing homes' performance of resident-centered care using management technology and data warehousing.

Data Mining

Data mining uses both exploratory and confirmatory statistical techniques to translate masses of raw data into valuable information for clinical and managerial decisions (Wan, 2006). Data mining in long-term care research could play an important role for quality improvement in a variety of areas. Significant areas for quality improvement include (1) understanding the patterns of care, (2) identifying root causes for clinical and managerial problems in the delivery of nursing home care, (3) profiling the best practice models in nursing homes, (4) establishing benchmarks that identify strategic directions for optimizing continuous improvement of care, and (5) differentiating the mechanisms for improving both nursing home care and nursing home management. A prime example is the application of a predictor tree analysis (see www. dtreg.com for details and exemplars). A predictor tree, based on analysis of variance (ANOVA), identifies factors that delineate either mutually exclusive or homogeneous subgroups of nursing homes that have different performance levels. Then specific predictor variables can be introduced to account for the variability in an outcome (e.g., resident's functional status) or in a performance indicator (e.g., technical efficiency) in each subgroup. The advantages of this two-tiered approach to data mining are (1) the ability to formulate a series of subgroups with different performance levels or outcomes, (2) the ability to specify predictive variables that can account for the variability in the performance level(s), and (3) the ability to develop managerial or clinical intervention strategies targeting a specific group of nursing homes to improve their quality of care.

Confirmatory Statistical Analysis

Confirmatory statistical analysis applies multivariate statistical methods, such as structural equation modeling (SEM), to validate or confirm a theoretically constructed model, as documented in our previous work (see Wan, 2002; Wan,

Zhang, and Unruh, 2006; Zhang, Unruh, and Wan, 2008). This modeling approach often uses latent variables, particularly for the subjectively reported and objectively assessed quality of care in nursing homes. The measurement model of the theoretical constructs is established and evaluated to determine the validity and reliability of the measurement instrument(s) used. Then functional or causal relationships among the study variables are evaluated in a structured equation model to assess their "goodness-of-fit" to the data gathered from the field study. Key examples of such measurement include the quality of nursing care (Wan, Zhang, and Unruh, 2006; Zhang and Wan, 2007), resident outcomes (Wan, Zhang, and Unruh, 2006), service scope expansion and rehabilitation (Murray et al., 2003), the effects of ownership on the quality of care (Zhao et al., 2009), and the effects of staffing on the quality of care in nursing homes (Konetzka, Stearns, and Park, 2008).

Based on Bayesian probability theory, Bayesian networks generate estimated probability distributions of unknown variables (such as the quality of care) from known probabilistic associations among multiple indicators of the structure, process, and outcome aspects of the quality of care in nursing homes (Goodson, Jang, and Rantz, 2008). This approach is similar to the development of structural equation modeling for portraying the structural relationships among study variables. The estimated joint probability distributions of quality indicators could be calculated from a product of conditional probabilities. Thus, statistical inferences can be drawn from known or measurable elements of quality indicators. In addition, the large data sets could be partitioned into subsets or subsamples so that the proposed model could be further validated or replicated in the subset or training data set.

Simulation and Optimization Methods

Simulation and optimization methods should play an important role in research on nursing home care. Researchers should build interfaces between analytical modeling and operations research. For instance, data envelopment analysis (DEA) should be applied to identify the best practice(s) in nursing homes and to suggest potential avenues for improving both the efficiency and the quality of nursing home care (Zhang, Wan and Unruh, 2008). Another example is the application of econometrics (statistical methods for examining economic data and issues) to simulate nurse staffing and related factors influencing the quality of care in nursing homes (Konetzka, Stearns, and Park, 2008). Graphics-user interface (GUI) presentations should be developed so that simulated results can guide managerial decisions. An example is the executive decision support system we developed to simulate how nursing home managers or executives can improve performance and the quality of care if they are willing to change operational management strategies, for example, by altering staff mix.

Translational Research

Translational research aims to convert scientific knowledge into practice, as in the design and evaluation of management interventions for nursing homes. With the assistance of information and communication technology, executives and other decision makers can rely on evidence-based knowledge to improve the efficiency, effectiveness, and quality of nursing home care. Unfortunately, state and federal agencies have not invested resources to launch or implement any sort of translational research on nursing home care.

The most important use of information and communication technology in nursing homes is to enhance resident-centered care and thus improve the quality of care. The National Commission for Quality Long-Term Care—an independent organization working to improve long-term care in the United States—strongly urges that patients' rights and patients' perspectives be considered in the evaluation and monitoring of the quality of care (National Commission for Quality Long-Term Care, 2008).

The Evidence-Based Modeling Approach

Evidence-based modeling and simulation of nursing home care and management is an important approach to improving overall care and quality. That process begins by a formulation of the study problem, guided by a theoretically informed framework to specify the inter-relationships among study variables. The analytical model is then specified and subsequently built iteratively with testable hypotheses. The analytical model serves as the basis for designing an empirical study that can, in turn, launch the construction of confirmatory statistical models. The measurement models and the causal models are developed and validated, and those results form the foundation and constraints for simulation and multivariate optimization modeling. Thus, a decision support system for managerial operations is formulated and can be further tested. The simulation is run and evaluated as a valid representation of the real-world system. Once that final validation is complete, the simulation model may be used to assess the real-world system and prescribe changes to improve the quality of

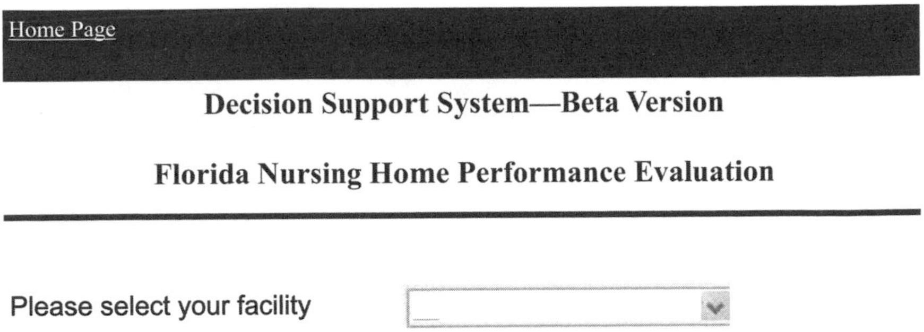

Home Page

Decision Support System—Beta Version

Florida Nursing Home Performance Evaluation

Please select your facility

Figure 8.4. Performance Evaluation of Florida Nursing Homes

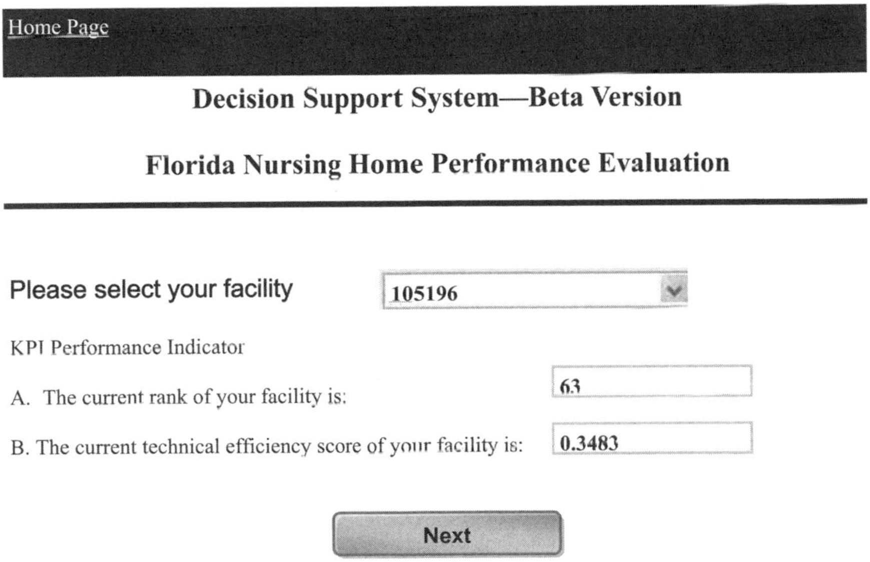

Home Page

Decision Support System—Beta Version

Florida Nursing Home Performance Evaluation

Please select your facility   105196

KPI Performance Indicator

A. The current rank of your facility is: 63

B. The current technical efficiency score of your facility is: 0.3483

Next

Figure 8.5. Technical Efficiency Score and Ranking for a Facility

care in nursing homes. In other words, the injection of artificial data simulating changes in input variables into the validated model for better performance is used to guide nursing home executives' decisions about improving the quality of the care they provide. Empirical examples illustrating the intricacy of such applied health care informatics research with emphasis on comparative effectiveness can be found in studies on nursing home management research

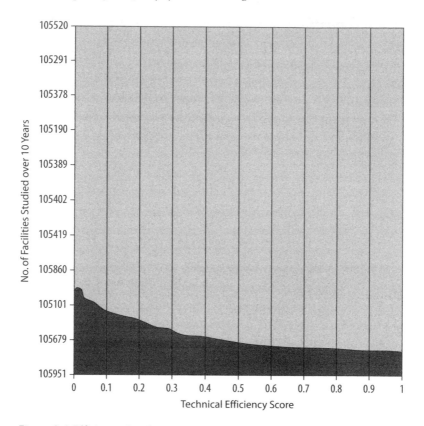

Figure 8.6. Efficiency Graph

(Zhang, Unruh, and Wan, 2008), nursing care staffing (Zhang et al, 2006) and the integration of information systems (Lee and Wan, 2002).

An example of an executive decision support system designed for nursing homes is described next. Based on the efficiency analysis of nursing homes in Florida, we performed an input-oriented Variable Returned to Scale (VRS) assumption in the DEA to include three input variables: (1) expenses of general services, (2) expenses of routine services, and (3) expenses of ancillary services—and three output variables: (1) skilled nursing inpatient days, (2) intermediate nursing inpatient days, and (3) other long-term care patient days. A graphic-user interface computing output is formulated in the following three steps: (1) enter the nursing home ID number in figure 8.4; (2) rank the facility based on the technical efficiency score for this facility in figure 8.5; and (3) show an efficiency graph with a different facility that has relatively poor performance in

Decision Support System—Beta Version

Florida Nursing Home Performance Evaluation

Your Facility is: 105198

The decision support system calculates the optimal improvement based on the slack of the current input variables (eg. with an input oriented efficiency model). Please change the optimal improvement to the desired improvement, for each of the three inputs and click the submit button to receive a new analysis of your facility.

A positive slack indicates that the expenses need to be reduced and the vice versa.

	Current Input	Slack	Optimal Input Improvement (In Percentage)
Expenses of general services	5054627.53	243481.31	4.62
Expenses of routine services	3456882.26	0	0
Expenses of ancillary services	838266.45	189670.36	22.55

	Current Output	Slack
Skilled nursing inpatient days	6341	0
Intermediate nursing inpatient days	58218	0
Other long term care inpatient days	0	0

Please input your email ID. (Analysis results
Will be emailed to the specified email ID.)

Submit

Figure 8.7 Decision Support System of Florida Nursing Home Performance Evaluation

figure 8.6. For illustrative purposes, we demonstrate the process for a facility (using ID# 105198) and use DEA to optimize the performance by altering the input variables to improve its ranking in figure 8.7.

Conclusion

Information technology, especially ehealth Web sites such as WebMD.com, as well as the Teaching Nursing Home program for teaching the essentials of nursing home care, can be useful resources in enhancing care and interventions in nursing home settings.

Informatics research in nursing homes is an interdisciplinary field that draws on knowledge from information, cognition management, computing, and communication sciences. Evidence-based informatics studies information science as it applies to nursing home management, compiling, managing, and processing data and information to help improve nursing home performance, including the quality of care. It is widely recognized, however, that the use of health information technology in nursing homes is underused and underdeveloped. A resident-centered, IT-based network should be built that can provide vital information at the point of care to improve residents' quality of care and outcomes. Although the empirical research on nursing home management is timely, the future of informatics research and development depends on transforming such knowledge into management and clinical practices. For instance, translational research should generate evidence-based knowledge to guide the development and implementation of consumer-oriented health IT to be embedded in hand-held devices (e.g., iphones). The needed step forward is to promote research activities with massive clinical and administrative data. This is a necessary and fundamental step toward achieving a better understanding of how clinical and managerial interventions affect resident outcomes. The ensuing development of evidence-based decision support systems, with a comparative perspective in both effectiveness and efficiency, should help to improve the quality of care in nursing homes, as informatics research guides the future delivery system. The elements in such a future delivery system will include services such as ehealth (virtual health mechanisms for educating nursing home residents) and syndromic surveillance (IT monitoring and tracking of the sources of the acute infections frequently threatening nursing home residents). Then perhaps improvement in nursing home care may finally appear on the horizon.

Synthesis, Prospects, and Future Directions

Synthesis

In this volume, we set out to accomplish a comprehensive analysis of the issues in the quality of care found in nursing homes across the United States. The overarching goal was to provide evidence-based approaches to improving the quality of nursing home care. We now conclude by reviewing the topics addressed.

In the introduction, a detailed discussion introduced nursing homes: what they are, how they have developed, and where they now stand. This historical information and the references for the development of nursing homes provide a starting point for understanding these complex and interdependent institutional, health care and medical systems.

Chapter 1 broadly laid out the quality of care in nursing homes. Definitions were provided for the quality of care and what it means in the nursing home environment. Quality of care was viewed from different perspectives including how staff interpersonal skills can affect resident quality of life (Barry, Brannon, and Mor, 2005). Statistical data revealed quantitative and qualitative disparities in care across different nursing homes, the ethnic groups they serve, and their urban and rural locations. The vast and diverse spectrum of care—depending on the location, racial or ethnic groups (Mor et al., 2004; Angelelli, Grabowski, and Mor, 2006; Miller et al., 2006), and the range of available resources—demonstrates the inconsistencies, differences, and issues found in nursing home systems.

Chapter 2 provided information and a review of the literature on how the quality of care is measured in nursing homes across the United States. We examined the instruments that measure and evaluate the quality of care in nursing homes. OSCAR (the Online Survey Certification and Reporting) data network managed and updated by the Centers for Medicare and Medicaid Services (Grabowski, Angelelli, and Mor, 2004) is one such system from which measurement of the quality of care is frequently drawn. The structure-process-outcome (SPO) model is a framework for understanding how nursing homes operate and function either well or poorly, efficiently or inefficiently, and deliver adequate or inadequate care. Beyond this model as a tool to assess quality of care, multilevel confirmatory factor analysis, a statistical method of approaching measurement was explained and applied to panel data on nursing homes.

Chapter 3 addressed specific factors to consider when measuring the quality of care in nursing homes. Deficiency citations—accidents, poor housekeeping, pressure ulcers, and/or catheterizations of residents—are common indicators of deficient care. Staff size, mix, rotations, and competence were also explained as they relate to the quality of care in nursing homes. The people who care for the residents are crucial in determining the quality of care received. Resident integrity, which refers to a resident's general psychosocial status, is also an important aspect in understanding how individual residents perceive the quality of care they receive. The size of the nursing home—how many beds it has and the number of staff members—are also determining factors that affect the quality of care. Residents who have cognitive, psychological, and/or motor dysfunction are common in nursing homes (Mitchell et al., 2003). How staff manage such residents is a key indicator of the quality and level of care. Rural nursing homes were also singled out for discussion with regard to quality of care because they sometimes lack the resources that urban, metropolitan, or suburban nursing homes have.

Chapter 4 presented an in-depth analysis of the clinical problem of persistent deficiencies frequently cited in the quality-of-care review in nursing homes. Despite being classified as only a localized soft-tissue wound, pressure ulcers have many serious clinical complications and a negative social impact for patients. Identifying risk factors related to persistent deficiencies in treating pressure ulcers in nursing homes and providing evidence-based knowledge to prevent deficiencies from resurfacing are key steps to reducing the occurrence of pressure ulcers. However, few studies have examined the development of persistent deficiencies of pressure ulcers in nursing homes. This chapter examined organizational, management, aggregate residential, and market factors associated with persistent deficiency citations for pressure ulcers in nursing homes. We conducted a pooled cross-sectional analysis of data from 1997 to

2007 of all certified U.S. nursing homes. We used both OSCAR data and Area Resource File (ARF). In addition to clinical factors, organizational, management, and market risk factors are associated with the development of persistent deficiencies in the treatment of pressure ulcers. Comprehensive care planning, resident assessment, total nurse staffing, and market demand are all positively associated with fewer persistent deficiencies in the treatment of pressure ulcers. Our study shows that a multidisciplinary approach integrating clinical, organizational, management, and market strategies provides better interventions for persistent deficiencies of pressure ulcers. Future studies should examine the effectiveness of multidisciplinary interventions on other deficiency citations.

In chapter 5, the variation in residents' health care outcomes with respect to prevalent health conditions such as pressure ulcers, physical restraints, and use of catheters in nursing homes was investigated using longitudinal data and latent growth curve modeling. The effects of contextual characteristics and nursing-related factors on the overall quality improvement of resident outcomes, measured by a weighted index in incidents of pressure ulcers, physical restraints, and use of catheters in nursing homes, were analyzed by autoregressive latent trajectory modeling of panel data (1997–2003). Findings show that in the initial study period, nursing homes having smaller bed size, operating as for-profit institutions, caring for more Medicare recipients, having residents with lower acuity levels, being located in the region other than the South, having a high level of nurse staffing, and being certified with lower frequencies of nursing care deficiencies had better quality. The intercept factor, representing the baseline of quality, was well predicted by six of the eight contextual and facility characteristics variables, and the slope or change trajectory of quality was only weakly predicted by them. The improved quality in resident outcomes was associated with facilities having fewer nursing care deficiency citations than their counterparts.

Chapter 6 discussed in detail policies relating to minimum nursing home staff levels. For example, the Nursing Home Reform Act of 1987 that seeks to ensure the best resident care mandates that adequate staff be present. The definition of "adequate," however, is still in question. Increased scrutiny and monitoring by federal and state governments now exists, and penalties are called for when services in nursing homes fall short because of a lack of staff and when poor care results. The chapter's policy analysis examined the significance of the legal oversight that seeks to ensure the quality of care in nursing homes.

Chapter 7 explored the assessment of efficiency and its relationship to the quality of care in nursing homes. Efficiency is important in nursing home practices. Maximizing resources with as little waste as possible or using all resources to their optimal capacity is crucial when resources are limited. Not only are competence, experience, and knowledge of policies pivotal to the success of a nursing home, but so is efficiency. We analyzed both cross-sectional and longitudinal data associated with nursing home performance in two major domains: technical efficiency and quality efficiency. Each nursing home in Florida was ranked in terms of its performance measured by technical efficiency and quality efficiency. Then the potential efficiency and quality trade-off relationship was examined by cross-sectional analysis and longitudinal panel analysis.

Chapter 8 presented a new view of nursing home practice and effectiveness by looking at how technology can be integrated to improve the quality of care in nursing homes. Ehealth services such as WebMd.com and other Internet-based health sites are full of health care information that can facilitate and/or improve diagnoses, treatment, and care practices. We examined ways of using health informatics research and practice to improve the operation of nursing homes. We introduced the field of informatics research in health and elder care, strategies in nursing home informatics research, and specific analytical methods: data warehousing, data mining, confirmatory statistical analysis, simulation and optimization methods, translational research, and evidence-based modeling.

Chapter 8 offers ideas that can spawn future research for scholars and practitioners who concentrate on nursing homes. These ideas serve as future directions for readers, researchers, and nursing home personnel and/or staff members in this complex and important sector of society.

Prospects

Efforts have been made to improve the quality of care in nursing homes through government and private initiatives. It is timely to address critical issues pertaining to quality improvement through collaboration among multiple professionals (Holthaus, 2009; Stevenson and Mor, 2009), particularly in light of health reforms. Research on health services and informatics offers a usable, practice-based referential resource for issues about nursing home care. The systematic assessment and evaluation data on nursing home practice can portray the structural, process, and outcome aspects of the quality of care in nursing homes. The SPO model posits that resident outcomes are directly influenced by the process aspect of nursing home care, whereas the process of care is itself directly influenced by the structural aspect of care. In fact, empirical evidence even suggests that the structural aspect of care also directly influences residents' outcomes. Thus, nursing home research should seriously consider that the structural aspect of care exerts both direct and indirect effects on residents' outcomes.

Several theoretically informed frameworks have been applied in the investigation of nursing home care. The paramount theory in this realm of research is known as the resource dependency theory, formulated by Pfeffer and Salancik (1978). In an empirical study using this theory, Harrington, Swan, and Carillo (2007) analyzed environmental factors that affect organizational decisions in nursing home care. As they pointed out, nursing homes, like other health organizations, rely upon available resources in the environment and make accommodations with the environment in order to sustain their survival. Because many nursing home facilities rely especially on revenue from Medicaid and Medicare (Grabowski, Angelelli, and Mor, 2004; Harrington, Swan, and Carillo, 2007), organizational features mediate decisions within the organization. Organizational characteristics also determine nursing homes' capacity to respond to contingencies.

Another relevant theory applicable to nursing home care is institutional theory, coined by Selznick (1948). A study by Zhang and Wan (2007) notes that institutional theory explains how organizations respond to institutional pressures to become isomorphic in their structures or processes in order to gain legitimacy, resources, and stability. Institutional isomorphism is driven by "pressures from other organizations on which a focal organization is dependent and an organization's pressure to conform to the cultural expectations of the larger society," and by "professionalism and uncertainty" (Mizruchi and Fein, 1999, p. 657). In short, institutional isomorphism is driven by coercive, normative, and mimetic mechanisms (Zhang and Wan, 2007). More than other popular organizational theories, institutional theory is especially sensitive to organizations' responses to social pressures.

Zhang and Wan (2007) assert that institutional theory can be applied to testing institutional effects in nursing homes. Their 2007 study examined the effects of institutional mechanisms on the isomorphism of nursing homes' quality of care, and supported the focus of earlier researchers on the regulatory aspects of institutions.

Limited research in this field has applied multilevel modeling of the determinants of nursing home care. To understand the micro- and macro-level factors influencing the variation in the quality of nursing home care, one must include the personal (individual) and contextual (ecological) factors that will either facilitate or impede the delivery of a high quality of nursing home care. For example, when assessing health care outcomes, one should consider the residents' quality of life.

The challenges in standardizing measurement of the quality of care have been well documented in health services research (Zhang and Wan, 2007). The prospects for employing standardized and well-designed indicators of the quality of nursing home care have improved through the quality improvement initiatives of the Centers for Medicare and Medicaid Services (see www.cms.gov/medicaid). Our research shows that official databases such as MDS and OSCAR yield feasible sources of information about residents' outcomes in general. Nevertheless, it is highly desirable to establish condition-specific indicators of the quality of care.

Practice-based evaluation of nursing homes' quality of care is needed for public policy on improving their care to be able to target the critical factors involved. Especially, the trade-off between efficiency and the quality of nursing home care must be carefully studied. Achieving the most efficiency possible without jeopardizing the quality of care should be the guiding principle. To that end, both clinical and executive decision-support systems derived from evidence-based research should be formulated. Nursing home staff and managers could then rely on scientific information to improve both operational management, and the quality of care and residents' quality of life.

Future Directions

Identifying prospective ideas generated by research is a good way to identify new topics for future research. This book has surveyed many published concepts and trends that give rise to innovative ideas for scholarly research and publication.

To start, as we looked at the quality of care in nursing homes, we noted how interpersonal communication skills of the staff can significantly affect the integrity of residents. Future research might examine specific ways in which staff's interpersonal skills could be adapted and tailored to meet the specific needs of the residents. For example, in cases in which residents have a communication disorder such as aphasia as a result of a brain injury (i.e., stroke,

aneurysm, etc.) (Quilliam, Lapane, Eaton, and Mor, 2001), the speech therapists who may be the clinical staff in the nursing home can act not only as
therapists, but also as integrity stabilizers or managers for those residents. Understanding the key particular needs of each resident is crucial for achieving
satisfactory levels of integrity. That goal may require additional time and effort
from the nursing home staff as well as from outsourced contractors who period-
ically work in the nursing home (Bourbonniere et al., 2006). The results, however, might prove to be lower resident mortality as well as improvement in their
moods and behavior. Moreover, the improvement in the residents' condition
can improve the morale and motivational levels of the staff caring for them.
This area is ripe for further investigation (Breen et al., 2009). Furthermore,
research on nursing home culture change is critically needed (Grant, 2008;
Rahman and Schnelle, 2008). We advocate the use of resident-centered approach to improve communications, pay attention to residents' concerns, and
develop homelike dinning and personal care modalities in nursing home care.
However, more rigorous evaluation research is certainly needed in demonstrating the efficacy or comparative effectiveness of varying intervention strategies
for improving nursing home care.

Ensuring competence in nursing home staff members is crucial to serving
the quality needs of the residents. Competence also has an effect on the quality
and degree of service delivered to residents by the staff members. Because reimbursement from the government (through Medicaid and/or Medicare) has
a tremendous impact on the functionality of a nursing home, in terms of resources, maintenance, performance, etc., auditing personnel regularly may
prove to be valuable as a motivating mechanism to increase the quality in each
of these areas. If a nursing home has substantial deficiencies and is cited and
recognized for such, financial reimbursement from outside parties may be withdrawn, creating the possibility for the nursing home to plunge. Hence, exploring additional ways such as the pay-for-performance policy or the prognostic-
outcome based payment system to improve the functioning of nursing homes,
to ensure a continuous flow of income, and to maintain high quality of care for
residents is a crucial line of research. Furthermore, long-term care researchers
have to explore what works and what doesn't work in the context of clinical
practices, using the comparative effectiveness approach advocated by the Centers for Medicare and Medicaid Services, the Agency for Healthcare Research
and Quality, and the National Institutes of Health.

Technology offers boundless possibilities for improving the overall quality of care in nursing homes. The availability of "Nursing Home Compare" for nursing home quality through the CMS website (see www.cms.gov) offers useful information to enhance consumer choice. The star rankings on nursing home facilities could guide the further development and improvement of nursing home performance (Baier et al., 2009). The development of executive and clinical decision support systems for performance improvement is imperative if the nursing home system is to be optimized. Personal health records (PHRs) may eventually become standardized among residents and even the general population, allowing better management of medical histories and preventing the duplication of services. Those possibilities tie into both clinical and practical efficiency. In other words, having full medical information and history about a given resident within ready reach should facilitate better care. Along the same lines, ehealth services such as Medlineplus.gov can give the medical staff richer information to help them treat residents with complicated conditions. Such ehealth services on the Internet are user-friendly, rapidly delivering encyclopedias of medical knowledge that may be of critical aid in complex or unexpected incidents in nursing homes. Thus, the benefits of e-health in nursing home practices should be further explored.

Obtaining the informed consent of nursing home residents presents some challenges to healthcare delivery and the quality of care. Particularly for residents who lack the basic sensory skills to understand messages and for residents with varying degrees of cognitive dysfunction (Wu et al., 2005a), understanding informed consent or simply obtaining consent to specific care becomes especially precarious. Family members can certainly facilitate this process, but ascertaining what residents truly want or do not want, accept or reject, prefer or dislike can interfere with the goal of delivering the best care to them. Future research should examine this area more carefully, and develop solutions that are resident-centered and can uncover residents' wishes about their care when their own expression is compromised, incomprehensible, or unreasonable. In another endeavor, methods to reduce injuries or incorrect treatments resulting from negligence, omission of information, failure to fully communicate, or lack of resident involvement or understanding should be researched and put into practice.

An intriguing question that often arises in end-of-life discussions is why it is during the last six months of life that the greatest medical expenses are commonly incurred by nursing home residents or elderly adults. Why are fortunes expended within that time frame? It seems apparent to many commentators on this problem that as a resident's death becomes imminent, every strenuous (also expensive, invasive, and fruitlessly distressing to the resident) intervention is applied to stave off the clearly inevitable. The question then is whether managerial greed or physicians' psychology or both explains this. This is a question with serious practical implications, and requires further investigation. Could it be that the quality of care given to residents who appear to be failing in health diminishes because staff lose hope for them and thus dedicate fewer resources to sustaining life? If the quality of care languishes during that period, could it be that those residents suffer more accidents and injuries and thus incur mounting expenses? Any case seeking reasons that this period at the close of life generates enormous medical expenses is important.

Research on the quality of nursing home care could benefit from the use of randomized trial design to evaluate the effects of quality improvement interventions at both resident and nursing home levels. A systematic review of quality improvement efforts in nursing homes reveals that a very small number of studies have assessed intervention effects on resident outcomes (Alexander and Hearld, 2009). The effects of health information technology use by nursing home residents and managers remains to be scientifically evaluated although a few of randomized, controlled trials have been conducted, using computerized decision support to reduce potentially inappropriate prescriptions (Terrell et al., 2009), employing an educational intervention to reduce the use of physical restraints (Huizing et al., 2009), improving the process of pain management (Swafford et al., 2009), applying a behavioral intervention for depression (Meeks et al., 2008), and implementing transitional care management strategies for the quality improvement (Dedhia et al., 2009).

Long-term care research is a highly challenging subfield of health services research. We therefore are grateful for generous support from the National Institute of Nursing Research, the National Institutes of Health. The availability of administrative datasets from the Centers for Medicare and Medicaid Services enables us to explore the complex relationships of the contextual and organizational factors among nurse staffing, the quality of nursing care, and resident outcomes. Our work has now ventured into a new horizon that requires an interdisciplinary approach to practice-based research on nursing homes. With the assistance and resources of care management technology and informatics, the prospect of developing evidence-based models for improving the performance of care in nursing homes is promising.

Appendix
Helpful Websites for Clinical Knowledge Management and the Quality of Care

AARP Research Center
  www.aarp.org/research

Agency for Healthcare Research and Quality (AHRQ)
  www.ahcpr.gov/qual/errorsix.htm

American Health Quality Association (AHQA)
  www.ahqa.org

American Society for Healthcare Risk Management (ASHRM)
  www.ashrm.org/asp/home/home.asp

American Society of Health-System Pharmacists (ASHP)
  www.ashp.org

Anesthesia Patient Safety Foundation (APSF)
  www.gasnet.org/societies/apsf

Anonymous Critical Incidents Reporting System (CIRS)
  www.medana.unibas.ch/eng/CIRS/CIRS.htm

Australia Patient Safety Foundation (APSF)
  www.apsf.net.au

Center for Information Technology (CIT)
  www.cit.nih.gov/home.asp

Centers for Disease Control and Prevention
  www.cdc.gov

Centers for Medicare and Medicaid Services (CMS)
  www.cms.hhs.gov/home/asp

Commonwealth Fund
  www.commonwealthfund.org

Dartmouth Atlas of Healthcare
  www.dartmouthatlas.org

Florida Teaching Nursing Home (TNH)
  www.geriu.org

Health Grades
   www.healthgrades.com

Human Factors Research Technology Division (NASA)
   http://human-factors.arc.nasa.gov

Institute for Healthcare Improvement (IHI)
   www.ihi.org

Institute for Safe Medication Practices (ISMP)
   www.ismp.org

Joint Commission for the Accreditation of Healthcare Organizations (JCAHO)
   www.jcaho.org

Kaiser Family Foundation State Health Facts
   www.statehealthfacts.org

Long-Term Care Information
   www.longtermcareinfo.com

Long-Term Care Facts on Care in the U.S.
   LTCfocUS.org

Massachusetts Coalition for the Prevention of Medical Errors (MCPME)
   www.mhalink.org/mcpme/mcpme_welcome.htm

Medical Device Safety Reports (MDSR)
   www.mdsr.ecri.org/index.asp

Medical Group Management Association (MGMA)
   www.mgma.org

MedlinePlus
   www.medlineplus.gov

Medscape
   www.medscape.com

Mental Help Network
   www.mentalhelp.net

National Library of Medicine
   www.ncbi.nlm.nih.gov

National Institutes of Health
   www.nih.gov

National Patient Safety Foundation (NPSF)
   www.npsf.org

National Quality Forum (NQF)
   www.qualityforum.org

Risk Management Foundation of the Harvard Medical Institutions (RMF)
   www.rmf.harvard.edu

Statistical Methods: Statistical Process Control
   www.anu.edu.au/nceph/surfstat/surfstat-home/surfstat.html

Simulation Center for Crisis Management Training in Health Care
http://pkpd.icon.palo-alto.med.va.gov/simulator/simulator.htm

State Health Facts (SHF)
www.statehealthfacts.org

Talking Quality
www.talkingquality.gov

U.S. Food and Drug Administration–MEDWatch
www.fda.gov/medwatch

United States Pharmacopoeia (USP)
www.usp.org

Veterans Health Administration (VHA)
www.patientsafetycenter.com/Audrey.nelson/med.va.gov

WebMD.com
www.webmd.com

References

Aaronson, W. E., Zinn, J., and Rosko, M. 1994. Do for-profit and not-for-profit nursing homes behave differently? *The Gerontologist* 34, 775–86.

Alexander, J. A., and Hearld, L. R. 2009. What can we learn from quality improvement research? A critical review of research methods. *Medical Care Research and Review* 66(3), 235–71.

Anderson, R. I., Hobbs, B. K., Weeks, H. S., and Webb, J. R. 2005. Quality of care and nursing home cost-efficiency research. *Journal of Real Estate Literature* 13(3), 325–35.

Anderson, R. I., Lewis, D., and Webb, J. R. 1999. The efficiency of nursing home chains and the implications of non-profit status. *Journal of Real Estate Portfolio Management* 5(3), 235–45.

Angelelli, J., Grabowski, D. C., and Mor, V. 2006. Effect of educational level and minority status on nursing home choice after hospital discharge. *American Journal of Public Health* 96(7), 1249–53.

Arling, G., Karon, S., Sainfort, F., Zimmerman, D., and Ross, R. 1997. Risk adjustment of nursing home quality indicators. *The Gerontologist* 37(6), 757–66.

Arnold, E. C., and Boggs, K. U. 2006. *Interpersonal relationships: Professional communication skills for nurses.* St. Louis: Saunders Press.

Atchley, S. 1991. A time-ordered, systems approach to quality assurance in long-term care. *Journal of Applied Gerontology* 10(1), 19–34.

Baier, R., Butterfield, K., Patry, G., Harris, Y., and Gravenstein, S. 2009. Identifying star performers: The relationship between ambitious targets and nursing home quality improvement, *Journal of the American Geriatrics Society* 57(8), 1498–1503.

Barker, K. N., Flynn, E. A., Pepper, G. A., Bates, D. W., and Mikeal, R. L. 2002. Medication errors observed in 36 health care facilities. *Archives of Internal Medicine* 162, 1897–1903.

Barry, T. T., Brannon, D., and Mor, V. 2005. Nurse aide empowerment strategies and staff stability: Effects on nursing home resident outcomes. *Gerontologist* 45(3), 309–17.

Bassett, W. F. 2007. Medicaid's nursing home coverage and asset transfers. *Public Finance Review* 35(3), 414–39.

Bellow, N. M., and Halpin, H. A. 2008. MDS-based state Medicaid reimbursement and the ADL-decline quality indicator. *The Gerontologist* 48, 324–29.

Berlowitz, D. R., and Frantz, R. A. 2007. Implementing best practices in pressure ulcer care: The role of continuous quality improvement. *Journal of the American Director Association* 8, S37–41.

Berlowitz, D. R., Young, G. J., Hickey, E. C., Saliba, D., Mittman, B. S., Czarnowski, E., et al. 2003. Quality improvement implementation in the nursing home. *Health Services Research* 38, 65–83.

Biesanz, J., Deeb-Sossa, N., Papadekis, A., Bollen, K., and Curran, P. 2004. The role of coding time in estimating and interpreting growth curve models. *Psychological Methods* 9(1), 30–52.

Bliesmer, M. M., Smayling, M., Kane, R. L., and Shannon, I. 1998. The relationship between nursing staffing levels and nursing home outcomes. *Journal of Aging and Health* 10(3), 351–71.

Bolin, J. N., Phillips, C. D., and Hawes, C. 2006. Differences between newly admitted nursing home residents in rural and nonrural areas in a national sample. *The Gerontologist* 46(1), 33–41.

Bollen, K. A., and Curran, P. J. 2004. Autoregressive latent trajectory (ALT) models: A synthesis of two traditions. *Sociological Methods and Research* 32(3), 336–83.

Bourbonniere, M., Feng, Z., Intrator, O., Angelelli, J., Mor, V., and Zinn, J. 2006. The use of contract licensed nursing staff in U.S. nursing homes. *Medical Care Research and Review* 63(1), 88–109.

Braun, B. 1991. The effect of nursing home quality on patient outcome. *Journal of the American Geriatrics Society* 39(4), 329–38.

Breen, G. M., and Matusitz, J. 2007. An interpersonal examination of telemedicine: Applying relevant communication theories. *eHealth International Journal* 3(1), 18–23.

Breen, G. M., and Zhang, N. J. 2008. Introducing ehealth to nursing homes: Theoretical analysis of improving resident care. *Journal of Medical Systems* 32(2), 187–92.

Breen, G. M., Matusitz, J., and Wan, T. T. H. 2009. The use of public policy analysis to enhance the Nursing Home Reform Act of 1987. *Social Work in Health Care* 48(05), 505–18.

Breen, G. M., Wan, T. T. H., Zhang, N. J., Marathe, S. S., Seblega, B. K., and Paek, S. C. 2009. Improving doctor-patient communication: Examining innovative modalities *vis-à-vis* effective patient-centric care management technology. *Journal of Medical Systems* 33(2), 155–162.

Cashen, M. S., Dykes, P., and Gerber, B. 2004. eHealth technology and Internet resources: Barriers for vulnerable populations. *Journal of Cardiovascular Nursing* 19(3), 209–14.

Castle, N. G. 2000. Deficiency citations for physical restraint use in nursing homes. *Journal of Gerontology*, Series B, 55 (1), S33–40.

——. 2001. Innovation in nursing homes. *Gerontologist* 41, 161–72.

——. 2002. Nursing homes with persistent deficiency citations for physical restraint use. *Medical Care* 40(10), 868–78.

——. 2003a. Providing outcomes information to nursing homes: Can it improve quality of care? *The Gerontologist* 43(4), 483–92.

——. 2003b. Strategic groups and outcomes in nursing facilities. *Health Care Management Review* 28, 217–27.

——. 2009. The Nursing Home Compare report card: Consumers' use and understanding. *Journal of Aging and Social Policy* 21(2), 187–208.

Castle, N. G., and Engberg, J. 2007a. The influence of staffing characteristics on quality of care in nursing homes. *Health Services Research* 42, 1822–47.

——. 2007b. Nursing home deficiency citations for medication use. *Journal of Applied Gerontology* 26(2), 208–32.

Castle, N. G., and Fogel, B. 1998. Characteristics of nursing homes that are restraint free. *The Gerontologist* 38(2), 181–88.

——. 2002. Professional association membership by nursing facility administrators and quality of care. *Health Care Management Review* 27, 7–17.

Centers for Medicare and Medicaid Services. 2009a. *Nursing Home Compare*. Retrieved March 15, 2009, from .www.medicare.gov/NHcompare/home.asp.

——. 2009b. *Special Focus Facility Initiative*. Retrieved March 15, 2009, from www.cms .hhs.gov/certificationandcomplianc/downloads/sfflist.pdf.

Charnes, A., Cooper, W. W., and Rhodes, E. 1978. Measuring the efficiency of decision making units. *European Journal of Operational Research* 2, 429.

Cho, S. 2001. Nurse staffing and adverse patient outcomes: A systems approach. *Nursing Outlook* 49(2), 78–85.

Clark, L., Jones, K., and Pennington, K. 2004. Pain assessment practices with nursing home residents. *Western Journal of Nursing Research* 26(7), 733–50.

Clay, K. S. 2007. Under pressure: Why can't SNFs cut pressure ulcer occurrence? *Contemporary Long Term Care* 30(2), 18–25.

Coburn, A. F., and Bolda, E. 1999. The rural elderly in long-term care. In T. Ricketts (Ed.), *Rural health in the U.S.* (pp. 65–89). New York: Oxford University Press.

Coburn, A. F., Bolda, E. J., and Keith, R. G. 2003. Variations in nursing home discharge rates for urban and rural nursing facility residents with hip fracture. *Journal of Rural Health* 19(2), 148–55.

Cohen, J. W., and Spector, W. D. 1996. The effect of Medicaid reimbursement on quality of care in nursing homes. *Journal of Health Economics* 15, 23–48.

Coward, R. T., Duncan, R. P., and Freudenberger, K. M. 1994. Residential differences in the use of formal services prior to entering a nursing home. *The Gerontologist* 34, 44–49.

Coward, R. T., Duncan, R. P., and Netzer, J. K. 1993. The availability of health care resources for elders living in nonmetropolitan persistent low-income counties in the south. *Journal of Applied Gerontology* 12(3), 368–87.

Cowles Research Group. 2005. Retrieved July 20, 2009, from www.longtermcareinfo .com/crg/about_oscar.html.

Davis, F. D. 1989. Perceived usefulness, perceived ease of use, and user acceptance of information technology. *Management Information Systems Quarterly* 13(3), 319–39.

Dedhia, F., Kravet, S., Bulger, J., Hinson, T., Sridharan, A., Kolodner, K., Wright, S., and Howell, E. 2009. A quality improvement intervention to facilitate the transition of older adults from three hospitals back to their homes. *Journal of American Geriatrics Society* 57, 1540–46.

Degenholtz, H.B., Rosen, J., Castle, N., Mittal, V., and Liu, D. 2008. The association between changes in health status and nursing home resident quality of life. *The Gerontologist* 48, 584–92.

Dellefield, M. E. 2006. Organizational correlates of the risk-adjusted pressure ulcer prevalence and subsequent survey deficiency citation in California nursing homes. *Research in Nursing and Health* 29, 345–58.

Donabedian, A. 1966. Evaluating the quality of medical care. *Milbank Memorial Fund Quarterly* 54(3), 166–206.

———. 1988. The quality of care: How can it be assessed? *Journal of American Medical Association* 260(12), 1743–48.

Elwell, F. 1984. The effects of ownership on institutional services. *The Gerontologist* 24, 77–83.

Feng, Z., Grabowski, D. C., Intrator, O., and Mor, V. 2006. The effect of state Medicaid case-mix payment on nursing home resident acuity. *Health Services Research* 41(4), 1317–36.

Ferrer, E., Hamagami, F., and McArdle, J. 2004. Modeling latent growth curves with incomplete data using different types of structural equation modeling and multilevel software. *Structural Equation Modeling* 11(3), 452–83.

Forbes-Thompson, S., and Gessert, C. E. 2006. Nursing homes and suffering: Part of the problem or part of the solution? *Journal of Applied Gerontology* 25(3), 234–51.

Fottler, M. 1987. Health care organizational performance: Present and future research. *Journal of Management* 13(2), 367–91.

Gage, B. 1999. Impact of the BBA on post-acute utilization. *Health Care Finance Review* 20(4), 103–26.

Gessert, C. E., and Calkins, D. R. 2001. Rural-urban differences in end-of-life care: The use of feeding tubes. *Journal of Rural Health* 17(1), 16–24.

Gessert, C. E., Haller, I. V., Kane, R. L., and Degenholtz, H. 2006. Rural-urban differences in medical care for nursing homes residents with severe dementia at the end of life. *Journal of the American Geriatrics Society* 54, 1199–1205.

Glass, A. 1991. Nursing home quality: A framework for analysis. *Journal of Applied Gerontology* 10(1), 5–18.

Goodhue, D. L., and Thompson, R. L. 1995. Task technology fit and individual performance. *Management Information Systems Quarterly* 19(2), 213–36.

Goodson, J., Jang, W., and Rantz, M. 2008. Nursing home care quality: From a Bayesian Network Approach. *The Gerontologist* 48(3), 338–48.

Gorecki, C., Brown, J. M., Nelson, E. A., Briggs, M., Schoonhoven, L., Dealey, C., Defloor, T., and Nixon, J. 2009. Impact of pressure ulcers on quality of life in older patients: A systematic review. *Journal of the American Geriatrics Society* 57(7), 1175–83.

Grabowski, D. C. 2001. Medicaid reimbursement and the quality of nursing home care. *Journal of Health Economics* 20, 549–69.

———. 2004. The admission of blacks to high-deficiency nursing homes. *Medical Care* 42(5), 456–64.

Grabowski, D. C., Angelelli, J. J., and Mor, V. 2004. Medicaid payment and risk-adjusted nursing home quality measures. *Health Affairs* 23(5), 243–52.

Grabowski, D. C., and Castle, N. G. 2004. Nursing homes with persistent high and low quality. *Medical Care Research and Review* 61(1), 89–115.

Grabowski, D. C., Feng, Z., Intrator, O., and Mor, V. 2004. Recent trends in state nursing home payment policies. *Health Affairs (Millwood)*, Suppl. Web Exclusives: W4-363-73.

Grabowski, D. C., and Stevenson, D. G. 2008. Ownership conversions and nursing home performance. *Health Services* Research 43, 1184–1203.

Granerud, A., and Severinsson, E. 2003. Preserving integrity: Experiences of people with mental health problems living in their own home in a new neighborhood. *Nursing Ethics* 10, 602–13.

Grant, L. A. 2008. *Culture change in a for-profit nursing home chain: An evaluation.* New York: Commonwealth Fund.

Greene, V. L., and Monahan, D. J. 1981. Structural and operational factors affecting quality of patient care in nursing homes. *Public Policy* 29(4), 399–415.

Gustafson, D. H., Sainfort, F., Van Konigsveld, R., and Zimmerman, D. R. 1990. The quality assessment index for measuring nursing home quality. *Health Services Research* 25(1), 97–127.

Handler, S. M., Wright, R. M., Ruby, C. M., and Hanlon, J. T. 2006. Epidemiology of medication-related adverse events in nursing homes. *American Journal of Geriatric Pharmacotherapy* 4, 264–72.

Harrington, C. 2001a. Nursing facility staffing policy: A case study for political change. *Policy, Politics, and Nursing Practice* 2(2), 117–27.

———. 2001b. Residential nursing facilities in the United States. *British Medical Journal* 323, 507–10.

Harrington, C., and Millman, M. 2001. *Nursing home staffing standards in state statutes and regulations*. Report prepared for the Henry J. Kaiser Family Foundation, Department of Social and Behavioral Sciences, University of California, San Francisco.

Harrington, C., and Swan, J. H. 2003. Nursing home staffing, turnover, and case mix. *Medical Care Research and Review* 60(3), 366–92.

Harrington, C., Carillo, H., and Blank, B. 2008. *Nursing facilities, staffing, residents, and facility deficiencies, 2001 through 2007*. Report published by the Department of Social and Behavioral Sciences, University of California, San Francisco. September.

Harrington, C., Swan, J. H., and Carillo, H. 2007. Nurse staffing levels and Medicaid reimbursement rates in nursing facilities. *Health Services Research* 42 (3), 1105-29.

Harrington, C., Kovner, C., Mezey, M., Kayser-Jones, J., Burger, S., and Mohler, M. 2000a. Experts recommend minimum nurse staffing standards for nursing facilities in the United States. *The Gerontologist* 40(1), 5–16.

Harrington, C., Zimmerman, D., Karon, S., Robinson, J., and Beutel, P. 2000b. Nursing home staffing and its relationship to deficiencies. *Journal of Gerontology* 55(5), 278–87.

Harrington, C., Woolhandler, S., Mullan, J., Carrillo, H., and Himmelstein, D. U. 2001. Does investor ownership of nursing homes compromise the quality of care? *American Journal of Public Health* 91(9), 1452–55.

Harris, Y., and Clauser, S. B. 2002. Achieving improvement through nursing home quality measurement. *Health Care Financing Review* 23(4), 5–9.

Hendrix, T. J., and Foreman, S. E. 2001. Optimal long-term care nurse-staffing levels. *Nursing Economics* 19(4), 164–75.

Hillmer, M. P., Wodchis, W. P., Gill, S. S., Anderson, G. M., and Rochon, P. A. 2005. Nursing home profit status and quality of care: Is there any evidence of an association? *Medical Care Research and Review* 62(2), 139–66.

Holthaus, M. 2009. Long-term care: A test bed for coming reform. *Geriatrics* 64(7), 7–8.

Hu, P. J., Chau, P. Y., Sheng, O. R., and Tam, K. Y. 1999. Examining the technology acceptance model using physician acceptance of telemedicine technology. *Journal of Management Information Systems* 16(2), 91–112.

Hughes, C. M., Lapane, K. L., and Mor, V. 2000. Influence of facility characteristics on use of antipsychotic medications in nursing homes. *Medical Care* 38(12), 1164–73.

Huizing, A. R., Hamers, J. P. H., Gulpers, M. J. M., and Berger, M. P. 2009. A cluster-randomized trial of an educational intervention to reduce the use of physical restraints with psychogeriatric nursing home residents. *Journal of American Geriatrics Society* 57(7), 1139–1148.

Institute of Medicine. 1986. *Improving the quality of care in nursing homes.* Washington, D.C.: National Academy Press.

——. 1996. *Nursing staff in hospitals and nursing homes: Is it adequate?* Washington, D.C.: National Academy of Sciences.

——. 2001. *Crossing the quality chasm: a new health system for the twenty-first century.* Washington, D.C.: National Academy Press.

Intrator, O., Feng, Z., Mor, V., Gifford, D., Bourbonniere, M., and Zinn, J. 2005. The employment of nurse practitioners and physician assistants in U.S. nursing homes. *The Gerontologist* 45(4), 486–95.

Jervis, L. L., and Manson, S. M. 2007. Cognitive impairment, psychiatric disorders, and problematic behaviors in a tribal nursing home. *Journal of Aging and Health* 19(2), 260–74.

Johnson, C. E., Dobalian, A., Burkhard, J., Hedgecock, D. K., and Harman, J. 2004. Predicting lawsuits against nursing homes in the United States, 1997–2001. *Health Services Research* 39(6 Pt 1), 1713–31.

Joint Commission on Accreditation of Healthcare Organizations. 2002. Nursing shortage poses serious health care risk. Expert panel offers solutions to national health care crisis. News release, August 7.

Kaiser Family Foundation. 2009. The Top Ten Deficiencies in U.S. Nursing Homes, 2005. Retrieved on July 20, 2009, from www.statehealthfacts.org/comparemaptable.jsp?ind=419&cat=8.

Kane, R. A., and Kane, R. L. 1988. Long-term care: Variations on a quality assurance theme. *Inquiry* 25, 132–46.

Kelly, C. M., Liebig, P. S., and Edwards, L. J. 2008. Nursing home deficiencies: An exploratory study of interstate variations in regulatory activity. *Journal of Aging and Social Policy* 20(4), 398–413.

Kihlgren, M., Hallgren, A., and Norberg, A. 1994. Integrity promoting care of demented patients: Patterns of interaction during morning care. *International Journal of Aging and Human Development* 39(4), 303–19.

Kim, H., Harrington, C., and Greene, W. H. 2009. Registered nurse staffing mix and quality of care in nursing homes: A longitudinal analysis. *The Gerontologist* 49(1), 81–90.

Knox, K. J., Blankmeyer, E. C., and Stutzman, J. R. 2001. The efficiency of nursing home chains and the implications of nonprofit status: A comment. *Journal of Real Estate Portfolio Management* 7(2), 177–82.

Konetzka, R. T., Stearns, S. C., and Park, J. 2008. The staffing-outcomes relationship in nursing homes. *Health Services Research* 43(3), 1025–42.

Konetzka, R. T., Yi, D., Norton, E. C., and Kilpatrick, K. E. 2004. Effects of Medicare payment changes on nursing home staffing and deficiencies. *Health Services Research* 39(3), 463–88.

Kramer, A. M., and Fish, R. 2001. The relationship between nurse staffing levels and the quality of nursing home care. In ABT Associates, *Appropriateness of minimum nurse staffing ratios in nursing homes: Phase II final report*, December 2001.

Kuhn, B. A., and Coulter, S. J. 1992. Balancing the pressure ulcer cost and quality equation. *Nursing Economics* 10, 353–59.

Kumlien, S., and Axelsson, K. 2002. Stroke patients in nursing homes: Eating, feeding, nutrition, and related care. *Journal of Clinical Nursing* 11(4), 498–509.

Lakey, S. L., Gray, S. L., Sales, A., Sullivan, J., and Hendrick, S. C. 2006. Psychotropic use in community residential care facilities: A prospective cohort study. *American Journal of Geriatric Pharmacotherapy* 4, 227–35.

Lawton, M. P. 1997. Positive and negative affective states among older people in long-term care. In R. L. Rubinstein and M. P. Lawton (Eds.), *Depression in long-term and residential care* (pp. 29–54). New York: Springer.

Lee, K. S., and Wan, T. T. H. 2002. Effects of hospitals' structural clinical integration on efficiency and patient outcome. *Health Services Management Research* 15(4), 234–44.

Lee, R., Bott, M., Gajewski, B., and Taunton, R. L. 2009. Modeling efficiency at the process level: An examination of the care planning process in nursing homes. *Health Services Research* 44:15–32.

Levy, C. R., Fish, R., and Kramer, A. M. 2004. Site of death in the hospital versus nursing home of Medicare skilled nursing facility residents admitted under Medicare's Part A benefit. *Journal of American Geriatrics Society* 52, 1247–54.

Linn, M. W., Gurel, L., and Linn, B. S. 1977. Patient outcome as a measure of quality of nursing home care. *American Journal of Public Health* 67, 337–44.

Liperoti, R., Pedone, C., Lapane, K. L., Mor, V., Bernabei, R., and Gambassi, G. 2005. Venous thromboembolism among elderly patients treated with atypical and conventional antipsychotic agents. *Archive of Internal Medicine* 165(22), 2677–82.

Maas, M. L., Kelley, L. S., Park, M., and Specht, J. P. 2002. Issues in conducting research in nursing homes. *Western Journal of Nursing Research* 24(4), 373–89.

Mackenzie, C., and Lowit, A. 2007. Behavioral intervention effects in dysarthria following stroke: Communication effectiveness, intelligibility and dysarthria impact. *International Journal of Language and Communication Disorders* 42(2), 131–53.

Matusitz, J., and Breen, G. M. 2007. Telemedicine: Its effects on health communication. *Health Communication* 21(1), 73–83.

———. 2007. E-Health: A new kind of telemedicine. *Social Work in Public Health* 23(1), 95–113.

Meeks, S., Teri, L., Haitsma, K. V., and Looney, S. 2006. Increasing pleasant events in the nursing home. *Clinical Case Studies* 5(4), 287–304.

Meeks, S., Looney, S. W., Haitsma, K. V., and Teri, L. 2008. BE-ACTIV: A staff-assisted behavioral intervention for depression in nursing homes. *The Gerontologist* 48, 105–14.

Mezey, M. D., Mitty, E. L., and Burger, S. G. 2008. Rethinking teaching nursing homes: Potential for improving long-term care. *The Gerontologist* 48 (1), 8–15.

Miller, S. C., Papandonatos, G. D., Fennel, M., and Mor, V. 2006. Facility and county effects on racial differences in nursing home restraint and antipsychotic quality indicators. *Social Science and Medicine* 63(12), 3046–59.

Mitchell, S., Teno, J., Roy, J., Kabumoto, G., and Mor, V. 2003. Clinical and organizational factors associated with feeding tube use among nursing home residents with advanced cognitive impairment. *Journal of the American Medical Association* 290, 73–80.

Mitka, M. 2003. Telemedicine eyes for mental health services: Approach could widen access for older patients. *Journal of the American Medical Association* 290(14), 1842–43.

Mizruchi, M. S., and Fein, L. C. 1999. The social construction of organizational knowledge: A study of the uses of coercive, mimetic, and normative isomorphism. *Administrative Science Quarterly* 44, 653–83.

Mor, V. 2003. A comprehensive clinical assessment tool to inform policy and practice: Applications of the Minimum Data Set. *Medical Care* 42(4), 1–9.

———. 2005. Improving the quality of long-term care with better information. *Milbank Quarterly* 83(3), 333–64.

Mor, V., and Allen, S. 1987. *Hospice care systems: Structure, process, costs, and outcome.* New York: Springer.

Mor, V., Finne-Soveri, H., Hirdes, J., Gilgen, R., and DuPasquier, J.-N. 2009. Long term care quality monitoring using the Inter*RAI* common clinical assessment language. In P. C. Smith, E. Mossialos, S. Leatherman, S., and I. Papanicolas (Eds.), *Performance measurement for health system improvement: Experiences, challenges and prospect.* Cambridge University Press.

Mor, V., Zinn, J., Angelelli, J., Teno, J., and Miller, S. 2004. Driven to tiers: Socioeconomic and racial disparities in the quality of nursing home care. *Milbank Quarterly* 82(2), 227–56.

Morris, J., Moore, T., Jones, R., Mor, V., Angelelli, J., Berg, K., et al. 2002. *Validation of long-term and post-acute care quality indicators* (CMS contract No. 500-95-0062/T.O. #4).

Morris, J., Murphy, K., Mor, V., Berg, K., and Moore, T. 2003. Validation of long-term and post-acute care quality indicators. *CMS Report, Contract No: 500–95–0062.*

Mueller, C. 2000. A framework for nurse staffing in long-term care facilities. *Geriatric Nursing* 21(5), 262–67.

Mueller, C., Arling, G., Kane, R., Bershadksy, J., Holland, D., and Joy, A. 2006. Nursing home staffing standards: their relationship to nurse staffing levels. *The Gerontologist* 46, 74–80.

Mullan, J. T., and Harrington, C. 2001. Nursing home deficiencies in the United States: A confirmatory factor analysis. *Research on Aging* 23(5), 503–31.

Murray, P. K., Singer, M., Dawson, N. V., Thomas, C. L., and Cebul, R. D. 2003. Outcomes of rehabilitation services for nursing home residents. *Archives of Physical Medical Rehabilitation* 84, 1129–36.

Muthén, L. K., and Muthén, B. O. 1998. *Mplus user's guide: Statistical analysis with latent variables.* Los Angeles, CA: Muthén & Muthén.

National Association of Rural Health Clinics. 1998. *Understanding and working with managed care: A guide for rural providers.* Washington, D.C.: National Association of Rural Health Clinics.

National Commission for Quality Long-Term Care. 2008. *The commission.* Washington, D.C.: Author.

Nayar, P., and Ozcan, Y. A. 2008. Data envelopment analysis comparison of hospital efficiency and quality. *Journal of Medical Systems* 32(3), 193–99.

Newcomer, R., Swan, J., Karon, S., Bigelow, W., Harrington, C., and Zimmerman, D. 2001. Residential care supply and cognitive and physical problem case mix in nursing homes. *Journal of Aging and Health* 13(2), 217–47.

Nyman, J. A. 1988. Improving the quality of nursing home outcomes. Are adequacy- or incentive-oriented policies more effective? *Medical Care* 26(12), 1158–71.

———. 1989. Excess demand, consumer rationality, and the quality of care in regulated nursing homes. *Health Services Research* 24(1), 105–27.

Omnibus Budget Reconciliation Act of 1987. Pub L. No. 100-203, Subtitle C: Nursing Home Reform.

Ozcan, Y. A., Jiang, H. J., and Pai, C. W. 2000. Do primary care physicians or specialists provide more efficient care? *Health Services Management Research 13*, 90–96.

Ozcan, Y. A., Luke, R. D., and Haksever, C. 1992. Ownership and organizational performance: A comparison of technical efficiency across hospital types. *Medical Care 30*(9), 781–94.

Ozcan, Y. A., Wogen, S. E., and Mau, L. W. 1998. Efficiency evaluation of skilled nursing facilities. *Journal of Medical Systems 22*(4), 211–23.

Ozgen, H., and Ozcan, Y. A. 2004. Longitudinal analysis of efficiency in multiple output dialysis markets. *Health Care Management Sciences 7*(4), 253–61.

Park, J., and Stearns, S. C. 2009. Effects of state minimum staffing standards on nursing home staffing and quality of care. *Health Services Research 44*, 56–78.

Pfeffer, J., and Salancik, G. 1978. *The external control of organizations: A resource dependence perspective*. New York: Harper & Row.

Phillips, C. D., Chen, M., and Sherman, M. 2008. To what degree does provider performance affect a quality indicator? The case of nursing homes and ADL changes. *The Gerontologist 48*, 330–37.

Philips, C. D., Hawes, C., and Fries, B. E. 1993. Reducing the use of physical restraints in nursing homes: Will it increase costs? *American Journal of Public Health 83*, 342–48.

Porell, F., Caro, F., Silva, A., and Monane, M. 1998. A longitudinal analysis of nursing home outcomes. *Health Services Research 33*(4), 835–65.

Porras, J. 1987. *Stream analysis: A powerful way to diagnose and manage organizational change*. Reading, MA: Addison-Wesley.

Powell, W., and DiMaggio, P. 1991. *The new institutionalism in organizational analysis*. University of Chicago Press.

Powers, B. A. 2005. Everyday ethics in assisted living facilities: A framework for assessing resident-focused issues. *Journal of Gerontological Nursing 31*, 31–37.

Preston, J., Brown, F. W., and Hartley, B. 1992. Using telemedicine to improve health care in distant areas. *Hospital and Community Psychiatry 43*(1), 25–32.

Prins, P. D., and Henderickx, E. 2007. HRM effectiveness in older people's and nursing homes: The search for best quality practices. *Nonprofit and Voluntary Sector Quarterly 36*(4), 549–71.

Putnam, M., Tang, F., Brooks-Danso, A., Pickard, J., and Morrow-Howell, N. 2007. Professionals' beliefs about nursing home regulations in Missouri. *Journal of Applied Gerontology 26*(3), 290–304.

Quilliam, B. J., Lapane, K. L., Eaton, C. B., and Mor, V. 2001. Effect of antiplatelet and anticoagulant agents on risk of hospitalization for bleeding among a population of elderly nursing home stroke survivors. *Stroke 32*(10), 2299–2304.

Rahman, A. N., and Schnelle, J. F. 2008. The nursing home culture-change movement: Recent past, present, and future directions for research. *The Gerontologist 48*(2), 142–48.

Rantz, M., Zwygart-Stauffacher, M., Popejoy, L., Grando, V., Mehr, D., Hicks, L., Conn, V., Wipke-Tevis, D., Porter, R., Bostick, J., Maas, M., and Scott, J. 1999b. Nursing home care quality: A multidimensional theoretical model integrating the views of consumers and providers. *Journal of Nursing Care Quality 14*(1), 16–37.

Rantz, M. J., Popejoy, L., Petroski, G. F., Madsen, R. W., Mehr, D. R., Zwygart-Stauffacher, M., et al. 2001. Randomized clinical trial of a quality improvement intervention in nursing homes. *The Gerontologist 41*(4), 525–38.

Rantz, M. J., Popejoy, L., Zwygart-Stauffacher, M., Wipke-Tevis, D., and Grando, V. T. 1999a. Minimum Data Set and Resident Assessment Instrument. Can using standardized assessment improve clinical practice and outcomes of care? *Journal of Gerontological Nursing* 25(6), 35–43.

Rice, R. E., and Katz, J. E. 2001. *The internet and health communication: Experiences and expectations*. Thousand Oaks, CA: Sage Publications.

Robinson, J. P. 2000. Managing urinary incontinence in the nursing home: Residents' perspectives. *Journal of Advanced Nursing* 31, 68–77.

Rogers, C. 1997. Non-metro elders better off than metro elders on some measures, not on others. *Rural Conditions and Trends* 8(2), 52–59.

Rosen, E. 2000. The death of telemedicine? *Telemedicine Today* 8(1), 14–17.

Rosenman, R., Siddharthan, K., and Ahern, M. 1997. Output efficiency of health maintenance organizations in Florida. *Health Economics* 6, 295–302.

Sainfort, F., Ramsay, J., and Monato, H. 1995. Conceptual and methodological sources of variation in the measurement of nursing facility quality: An evaluation of 24 models and an empirical study. *Medical Care Research Review* 52(1), 60–87.

SAS User's Guide: Version 9 edition. Cary, NC: SAS Institute, Inc.

Schlenker, R. E., and Shaughnessy, P. W. 1996. The role of the rural hospital in long term care. In G. D. Rowles, J. E. Beaulieu, and W. W. Myers (Eds.), *Long-term care for the rural elderly: New directions in services, research, and policy* (pp. 132–55). New York: Springer Publishing.

Schnelle, J. F., Newman, D. R., and Fogarty, T. 1990a. Statistical quality control in nursing homes: assessment and management of chronic urinary incontinence. *Health Services Research* 25(4), 627–37.

———. 1990b. Management of patient continence in long-term care nursing facilities. *The Gerontologist* 30(3), 373–76.

Schnelle, J. F., Bates-Jensen, B. M. Levy-Storms, L. Grbic, V., Yoshii, J., Cadogan, M. P., and Simmons, S. F. 2004a. The Minimum Data Set prevalence of restraint quality indicator: does it reflect differences in care? *The Gerontologist* 44(2), 245–55.

Schnelle, J. F., Simmons, S. F., Harrington, C., Cadogan, M., Garcia, E., and Bates-Jensen, B. M. 2004b. Relationship of nursing home staffing to quality of care. *Health Services Research* 39, 225–50.

Scott-Cawiezell, J., Pepper, G. A., Madsen, R. W., Petroski, G., Vogelsmeier, A., and Zellmer, D. 2007. Nursing home error and level of staff credentials. *Clinical Nursing Research* 16(1), 72–78.

Seblega, B. K., Zhang, N. J., Unruh, L. Y., Breen, G. M., Paek, S. C., and Wan, T. T. H. 2010. Changes in nursing home staffing levels, 1997 to 2007. *Medical Care Research and Review* (in press).

Selznick, P. 1948. Foundations of the theory of organizations. *American Sociological Review* 13, 25–35.

Shah, A., Fennell, M., and Mor, V. 2001. Hospital diversification into long-term care. *Health Care Management Review* 26, 86–100.

Shaughnessy, P.W., Kramer, A.M., Hittle, D.F., and Steiner, J.F. 1995. Quality of care in teaching nursing homes: Findings and implications. *Health Care Financing Review* 16(4), 55–83.

Sloane, P. D., Miller, L. L., Mitchell, C. N., Rader, J., Swafford, K., and Hiattm, S. O. 2007. Provision of morning care to nursing home residents with dementia: Opportunity for improvement? *American Journal of Alzheimer's Disease and Other Dementias* 22(5), 369–77.

Smith, D. 1995. Pressure ulcers in the nursing home. *Annals of Internal Medicine* 123, 433–38.

Smyth, D. J. 1991. A model of quality changes in higher education. *Journal of Economic Behavior and Organization* 15, 151–57.

Spector, W., Selden, T., and Cohen, J. 1998. The impact of ownership type on nursing home outcomes. *Health Economics* 7(7), 639–53.

Spector, W. D., and Takada, H. A. 1991. Characteristics of nursing homes that affect resident outcomes. *Journal of Aging and Health* 3(4), 427–54.

Squillace, M. R., Remsburg, R. E., Harris-Kojetin, L. D., Bercovitz, A., Rosenoff, E., and Han, B. 2009. The national nursing assistant survey: Improving the evidence base for policy initiatives to strengthen the certified nursing assistant workforce. *The Gerontologist* 49(2), 185–97.

Stevenson, D. G. 2006. Nursing home consumer complaints and quality of care: A national view. *Medical Care Research and Review* 63(3), 347–68.

Stevenson, D. G., and Mor, V. 2009. Targeting nursing homes under the quality improvement organization program's 9th statement of work. *Journal of American Geriatrics Society* 57, 1678–84.

Stevenson, J., Beck, C., Heacock, P., Mercer, S., O'Sullivan, P., Hoskins, J., Doan, R., and Schnelle, J. 2000. A conceptual framework for achieving high-quality care in nursing homes. *Journal of Healthcare Quality* 22(4), 31–36.

Straker, J. 1999. *Reliability of OSCAR occupancy, census, and staff data: A comparison with the Ohio Department of Health Annual Survey of Long-Term Care Facilities.* Oxford, OH: Scripps Gerontology Center.

Street, R. L. 2001. Active patients as powerful communicators: The linguistic foundation of participation in health care. In W. P. Robinson (Ed.), *Handbook of language and social psychology* (pp. 541–60). Chichester: John Wiley.

Swafford, K. L., Miller, L. L., Tsai, P. F., Herr, K. A., and Ersek, M. 2009. Improving the process of pain care in nursing homes: A literature synthesis. *Journal of American Geriatrics Society* 57(6), 1080–87.

Swan, J., Harrington, C., Clemena, W., Pickard, R., Studer, L., and Dewit, S. 2000. Medicaid nursing facility reimbursement methods, 1979–1997. *Medical Care Research Review* 57(3), 361–78.

Teeri, S., Välimäki, M., Katajisto, J., and Leino-Kilpi, H. 2007. Maintaining the integrity of older patients in long-term institutions: Relatives' perceptions. *Journal of Clinical Nursing* 16(5), 918–27.

Temkin-Greener, H., Cai, S., Katz, P., Zhao, H., and Mukamel, D. B. 2009. Daily practice teams in nursing homes: Evidence from New York State. *The Gerontologist* 49(1), 68–80.

Terrell, K. M., Perkins, A. J., Dexter, P. R., Hui, S. L., Callahan, C. M., and Miller, D. K. 2009. Computerized support to reduce potentially inappropriate prescribing to older emergency department patients: A randomized, controlled trial. *Journal of American Geriatrics Society* 57, 1388–94.

Turnbull, G. 2000. Understanding the Balanced Budget Act of 1997. *Ostomy Wound Management* 46(1), 40–46.

Turner, J. W. 2003. Telemedicine: Expanding healthcare into virtual environments. In

T. L. Thompson, A. M. Dorsey, K. I. Miller, and R. Parrott (Eds.), *Handbook of health communication* (pp. 515–35). Mahwah, NJ: Lawrence Erlbaum Publishers.

Turner, J. W., Thomas, R. J., and Reinsch, N. L. 2004. Willingness to try a new communication technology: Perpetual factors and task situations in a health care context. *Journal of Business Communication* 41(1), 5–26.

Unruh, L., and Wan, T. T. H. 2004. A systems framework for evaluating nursing care quality in nursing homes. *Journal of Medical Systems* 28(2), 197–214.

Unruh, L., Zhang, N. J., and Wan, T. T. H. 2006. The impact of Medicare reimbursement changes on staffing and the quality of care in nursing homes. *International Journal of Public Policy* 1(4), 421–34.

Unützer, J., and Bruce, M. L. 2002. The elderly. *Mental Health Services Research* 4(4), 245–47.

U.S. Department of Health and Human Services. 1992. *Pressure ulcers in adults: Prediction and prevention* (Clinical Practice Guideline Number 3).Rockville, MD: Author.

———. 2004. *Register: HFS 132.45*. Madison: Author Press.

U.S. Department of Health and Human Services, Office of Inspector General. 1999. *Quality of care in nursing homes: An overview* (OEI-02-99-00060). Washington, D.C.: Author.

———. 2003. *Nursing home deficiency trends and survey and certification process consistency* (OEI-02-01-00600). March.

———. 2008. *Trends in nursing home deficiencies and complaints* (OEI-02-08-00140). September.

U.S. Department of Labor, Bureau of Labor Statistics. Employment in the health sector, 2000, *Current Population Survey: Employment and earnings*. January 2008.

U.S. General Accounting Office. 1999. *Nursing homes: Additional steps needed to strengthen enforcement of federal quality standards*. Washington, D.C.: Government Printing Office, GAO/HEHS-99–46.

———. 2005. *Nursing homes: Despite increased oversight, challenges remain in ensuring high-quality care and resident safety* (GAO-06-117). Washington, D.C.: General Accounting Office.

———. 2008. *Nursing homes: Federal monitoring surveys demonstrate continued understatement of serious care problems and CMS oversight weaknesses* (GAO-08-517). Washington, D.C.: General Accounting Office.

Vogelsmeier, A., Scott-Cawiezell, J., and Zellmer, D. 2007. Barriers to safe medication administration in the nursing home. *Journal of Gerontological Nursing* 33(4), 5–12.

Walley, T., and Scott, A. K. 1995. Prescribing in the elderly. *Postgraduate Medical Journal* 71(838), 466–71.

Walshe, K. 2001. Regulating U.S. nursing homes: Are we learning from experience? *Health Affairs* 20(6), 128–44.

Walshe, K., and Harrington, C. 2002. Regulation of nursing facilities in the United States: An analysis of resources and performance of state survey agencies. *The Gerontologist* 42, 475–86.

Wan, T. T. H. 2002. *Evidence-based health care management*. Norwell, MA: Kluwer Academic Publishers.

———. 2003. Nursing care quality in nursing homes: Cross-sectional versus longitudinal analysis. *Journal of Medical Systems* 27(3), 283–95.

———. 2006. Healthcare informatics research: From data to evidence-based practice. *Journal of Medical Systems* 30(1), 3–7.

Wan, T. T. H., and Connell, A. M. 2003. *Monitoring the quality of health care: Issues and scientific approaches.* Norwell, MA: Kluwer Academic Publishers.

Wan, T. T. H., and Lee, K. H. 2009. Healthcare informatics research. In R. M. Mullner (Ed.). *Encyclopedia of health services research,* Vol. 1, pp. 468–72. Thousand Oaks, Calif.: Sage Publications.

Wan, T. T. H., Zhang, N. J., and Unruh, L. 2006. Predictors of resident outcome improvement in nursing homes. *Western Journal of Nursing Research* 28(8), 974–93.

Wang, C. 2007. A pilot study of the perceived nursing home care needs instrument. *eHealth International Journal* 3(1), 10–17.

WebMD.com. 2008. About WebMD.com: Our products and services. WebMD Corporation, http://www.webmd.com/about-webmd-policies/default.htm?ss=ftr.

Weech-Maldonado, R., Shea, D., and Mor, V. 2006. The relationship between quality of care and costs in nursing homes. *American Journal of Medical Quality* 21(1), 40–48.

Wiener, J. M., Squillace, M. R., Anderson, W. L., and Khatutsky, G. 2009. Who do they stay: Job tenure among certified nursing assistants in nursing homes. *The Gerontologist* 49(2), 198–210.

Williams, C. L., and Tappen, R. M. 2007. Effect of exercise on mood in nursing home residents with Alzheimer's disease. *American Journal of Alzheimer's Disease and Other Dementias* 22(5), 389–97.

Wipke-Tevis, D., Williams, D., Rantz, M., Popejoy, L. L., Madsen, R. W., Petroski, G. F., et al. 2004. Nursing home quality and pressure ulcer prevention and management practices. *Journal of the American Geriatrics Society* 52, 583–88.

Wootton, R. 2001. Telemedicine. *British Medical Journal* 323, 557–60.

Wright, D. 1998. Telemedicine and developing countries. *Journal of Telemedicine and Telecare* 4(2), 2–37.

Wu, N., Miller, S. C., Lapane, K., Roy, J., and Mor, V. 2005a. Impact of cognitive function on assessments of nursing home residents' pain. *Medical Care* 43(9), 934–39.

———. 2005b. The quality of the quality indicator of pain derived from the Minimum Data Set. *Health Services Research* 40(4), 1197–1216.

Zhang, X., and Grabowski, D. C. 2004. Nursing home staffing and quality under the nursing home reform act. *The Gerontologist* 44 (1), 13–23.

Zhang, N. J., and Wan, T. T. H. 2005. The measurement of nursing home quality: Multilevel confirmatory factor analysis of panel data. *Journal of Medical Systems* 29(4), 401–11.

———. 2007. Effects of institutional mechanisms on nursing home quality. *Journal of Health and Human Services Administration* 29(4), 380–408.

Zhang, N. J., Unruh, L., and Wan, T. T. H. 2008. Has the Medicare prospective payment system led to increased nursing home efficiency? *Health Services Research* 43(3), 1043–61.

Zhang, N. J., Unruh, L., Liu, R., and Wan, T. T. H. 2006. Minimum nurse staffing ratios for nursing homes. *Nursing Economics* 24(2), 78–85.

Zhao, M., Oetjen, R. M., Nolin, J. M., and Carretta, H. J. 2010. Nursing home quality: Does financial performance matter? *International Journal of Public Policy* 5(2/3): 143–159.

Zimmerman, D. R., Karon, S. L., Arling, G., Clark, B. R., Collins, T., Ross, R., and Sainfort, F. 1995. Development and testing of nursing home quality indicators. *Health Care Finance Review* 16(4), p. 107.

Zinn, J., and Mor, V. 1998. Organizational structure and the delivery of primary care to older Americans. *Health Services Research* 33(2), 354–80.

Zinn, J., Mor, V., Intrator, O., Feng, Z., Angelelli, J., and Davis, J. 2003. The impact of the prospective payment system for skilled nursing facilities on therapy service provision: A transaction cost approach. *Health Services Research* 38(6), 1467-85.

Index

Page numbers followed by *t* refer to tables; page numbers followed by *f* refer to figures.

Abt Associates, Inc., 78–79
activities of daily living, 15, 17, 42, 62
acuity of residents: in pressure ulcer examination, 52, 54–55t, 56t, 107; as quality factor, 11; in resident outcome study, 62–63, 67, 68t, 72–73t, 74; rural nursing homes and, 14–15
African Americans, 13t, 13
age: as quality of care variable, 6; in resident outcome study, 62–64, 67, 68t, 72–73t, 74; rural nursing homes and, 14–16
Agency for Health Care Policy and Research, 57
allocative efficiency, 81
Alzheimer's disease, 42–43
American Indians, 13t, 13–14
aphasia, 43
Area Resource File (ARF), 10t, 49–50, 96–97, 107
Atchley structure-process-outcome model, 24

Balanced Budget Act (1997), 18, 26–27, 61–62, 89
Balanced Budget Reconciliation Act (1999), 18–19, 26–27, 62
Basset, W. F., 4
bed size: deficiency citations and, 36; as quality factor, 11; in resident outcome study, 62–64, 67, 68t, 72–73t, 74, 107
behavioral problems, 14, 42, 44
Benefits Improvement and Protection Act (2000), 18–19, 62
Berlowitz, D. R., 57
Blacks, 13t, 13
Bolda, E., 14

Bolin, J. N., 14
Bollen, K. A., 65
Braun, B., 61, 79–80
Breen, G. M., 2, 10, 90–93, 91–95
Brown, F. W., 91

Carillo, H., 109
Cashen, M. S., 12
Castle, N. G., 6, 36, 41, 57, 79
catheterization, 33–34, 63–64
Caucasians, 13
Center for Health Systems Research and Analysis, 9, 20
Centers for Medicare and Medicaid Services (CMS): certification and, 2, 20; deficiency penalties and, 50; incentive payments and, 89; Minimum Data Set (MDS) and, 1, 110; minimum nurse staffing and, 78–79, 80; on quality, 6–7, 34; report card system of, 5
certificates-of-need, 18, 63
Certified Nursing Assistants (CNAs), 1, 76–80
chain affiliation: efficiency and, 83; lawsuits and, 41; OSCAR data and, 21; percentages of, 4t, 4; in pressure ulcer examination, 51–52, 54–55t, 55, 56t; as quality factor, 11; in resident outcome study, 62–63, 67, 68t, 72–73t
Charnes, A., 84
CMS Special Focus Facility initiative, 50, 57
Coburn, A. F., 14
cognitive impairment, 14–15, 17, 42–44, 106
complaints, 2, 7–8

comprehensive care planning: and pressure ulcer examination, 47–48, 51, 53, 54–55t, 56t,
57, 107; staffing and, 9, 61, 79
consistency of care level, 6
contextual components, 27–28, 59–60, 61–63, 107
contractures, 34
Cooper, W. W., 84
cost efficiency, 84–85, 85f
costs, 2–5, 28, 47, 79, 91–92
Curran, P. J., 65

data mining, 96, 97f, 98, 108
data warehousing, 96–98, 97f, 108
Davis, F. D., 93
deficiencies, 4–5, 7, 9, 20, 33–34, 35t
deficiency citations: continued, 34; lawsuits and,
41; nursing home selection and, 19, 32; penalties for, 5; process measures and, 47; quality of
care measurement model and, 86; in resident
outcome study, 63–64, 67–73, 68t, 70f, 71f,
72–73t, 74–75; severity of, 58; top twenty, 48t;
tracked, 4–5, 9, 20
deficiency examination: discussion of, 57–58,
106–7; methodology of, 49–53; results of, 53,
54–55t, 55, 56t
dementia, 42, 44, 52
depression, 12, 40, 113
discharge rates, 61, 79, 80
Donabedian measurement model, 23–24, 25–
26, 60
do-not-resuscitate orders, 14
Dykes, P., 12

economic status, 14–16
efficiency: evidence-based modeling and, 102f,
102–4, 103f; factors influencing, 81–83; minimum staffing levels and, 76; quality of care
and, 107–8; types of, 81
ehealth, 90–95, 108
employment, 2–3, 3f
Engberg, J., 35, 36, 41, 79
ethnicity, 12–14, 13t, 105
evidence-based modeling, 100–104, 108
evidence-based research, 1, 5
expanded structure-process-outcome measurement model, 23f, 23, 27–31, 57, 60, 73
external factors, 18–19, 22, 26, 60–63, 81–82

facility characteristics, 62
facility-level measurement, 18, 73–74
facility size: efficiency and, 83, 84–85; in pressure ulcer examination, 51–52, 54–55t, 56t; in
proposed structure-process-outcome model,
28; and quality of care, 41, 106
fixed payments, 82
Florida Teaching Nursing Home program. *See*
Teaching Nursing Home program
Foreman, S. E., 9, 37, 79
Frantz, R. A., 57

gender, 2
General Accounting Office (GAO), 20, 22, 46
Gerber, B., 12
Glass structure-process-outcome model, 24
Goodson, J., 60
government regulation, 6, 18–19
Grabowski, D. C., 6, 12, 13, 37

Harrington, C., 9, 20, 31, 41, 78, 109
Hartley, B., 91
Hawes, C., 14
Health Care Financing Administration (HCFA), 20
Health Services Research, 4
Hendrix, T. J., 9, 37, 79
Hispanics, 13
hospice services, 44
hospital affiliation, 11, 14, 51–52, 54–55t, 56t
Hu, P. J., 93
Hughes, C. M., 41

incentive payments, 59, 82, 89
incontinence, 33, 52
Indian Health Service (IHS), 13–14
informatics research, 96–100, 97f, 101–3, 108
information technology, 90–95, 101–3, 108
institutional components, 27
institutional isomorphism, 109
institutional theory, 109
insurance coverage, 4, 14–16
isolation, 40–41

Jang, W., 60
Joint Commission on Accreditation of
Healthcare Organizations (JCAHO), 36
Journal of Medical Systems, 28

Kaiser Family Foundation, 34
Kane, R. A., 7
Kane, R. L., 7
Keith, R. G., 14

Lapane, K. L., 41
lawsuits, 41, 62
legislation: Balanced Budget Act, 18, 26–27, 61–62, 89; Balanced Budget Reconciliation Act, 18–19, 26–27, 62; Benefits Improvement and Protection Act, 18–19, 62; federal-level, 1, 18; Nursing Home Reform Act, 1, 42, 77, 80; Omnibus Budget Reconciliation Act, 20, 47, 77; and resident outcomes, 61–62
Lemke, S., 7
licensed practical nurses, 76–80
living wills, 14
location. *See* non-U.S. nursing homes; regional location; size, metropolitan
loneliness, 40–41

managed care organizations, 16
market competition, 54–55t, 56t, 81, 83, 107
market factors: and multi-level measurement models, 31–32; in pressure ulcer examination, 50, 53, 54–55t, 55, 56t, 57; and quality of care, 27, 62–63
Matusitz, J., 90–93
Mau, L. W., 83, 84
MDS. *See* Minimum Data Set (MDS)
measurement instruments, 17, 19–20, 105–6
Medicaid/Medicare: costs and, 3–4; in informatics research, 96–97; measurement models and, 17–18, 32; psychiatric care and, 42; rural nursing homes and, 14–15; state regulation and, 18
Medicaid/Medicare certification, 2, 9, 17–19, 77
Medicaid/Medicare reimbursements, 17–19, 36, 54–55t, 55, 56t, 109, 111
Medicaid percentage: deficiency citations and, 36; efficiency and, 83–85; in pressure ulcer examination, 51–52, 54–55t, 55, 56t; as quality factor, 6, 11; rural nursing homes and, 14–15
Medicare percentage, 63–64, 67, 68t, 70–71, 72–73t, 74, 84
Medicare prospective payment schedule, 18, 59, 62, 81–82

medication errors, 34–36
mental health, 12, 15, 40, 61
metropolitan size. *See* size, metropolitan
Minimum Data Set (MDS): certification and, 2; in informatics research, 96–97; multi-level measurement modeling and, 22; in nursing home research, 1, 8–9, 20
minimum staffing levels, 37–39, 76–80, 95, 107. *See also* nurse staffing; staff mix
Mitka, M., 92
Monato, H., 24, 28
mood disorders, 43
Moos, R. H., 7
Mor, V., 41
mortality rates, 6, 15, 34, 61, 79–80
Mueller measurement model, 25
Mullan, J. T., 9, 20, 31
multi-level measurement models, 22, 31–32, 106, 109–10
Multi-Phasic Environmental Assessment Procedure (MEAP), 7

National Commission for Quality Long-Term Care, 100
National Committee on Vital Health Statistics, 98
Nayer, P., 85
non-U.S. nursing homes, 95
nurse staffing: economic theory and, 37; efficiency and, 82–83; minimum levels of, 76–80; pressure ulcers and, 48–49, 51, 53, 57, 107; and quality of care, 11, 19, 36–39, 61, 79; and registered nurses (RNs), 7, 36, 76–80, 83; in resident outcome study, 63–64, 67–73, 68t, 70f, 71f, 72–73t, 74–75, 107; rural nursing homes and, 14–15. *See also* staff mix
nursing care adequacy, 86. *See also* deficiency citations
Nursing Economics, 38
nursing home care, 2, 6, 8–11, 108–10
Nursing Home Case Mix and Quality Demonstration, 9
Nursing Home Compare, 47, 58, 112
Nursing Home Reform Act (1987), 1, 42, 77, 80
nursing shortages, 19, 36–37
nutrition, 47, 51–52, 54t, 56t

occupancy rates, 51–52, 83, 84–85
Omnibus Budget Reconciliation Act (1987), 20, 47, 77
Online Survey, Certification, and Reporting (OS-CAR): in informatics research, 96–97; in nursing home research, 1, 8–10, 10t, 20–22, 106, 110; in pressure ulcer examination, 49–50, 107; in resident outcome study, 63–64
optimal nurse staffing levels, 79. *See also* nurse staffing; staff mix
organizational factors, 24–25, 36, 59–60
OSCAR. *See* Online Survey, Certification, and Reporting
outcome measures, 20, 23, 26, 60
ownership type: efficiency and, 82–83, 84; in expanded structure-process-outcome model, 28; lawsuits and, 41; percentages of, 4t, 4; in pressure ulcer examination, 51–52, 54–55t, 56t; as quality factor, 11; in resident outcome study, 62–63, 67, 68t, 72–73t, 74, 107
Ozcan, Y. A., 83, 84, 85

pain treatment, 42–44, 113
patient satisfaction, 34
payment mix: deficiency citations and, 36; efficiency and, 81, 83–85; in expanded structure-process-outcome model, 28; in pressure ulcer examination, 51–52, 54–55t, 56t; as quality factor, 11, 19; in resident outcome study, 62–65, 67, 68t, 70–71, 72–73t
Pfeffer, J., 109
Phillips, C. D., 14
Porras/Stevenson measurement model, 24–25
pressure ulcer examination, 57–58, 106–7; methodology of, 49–53; results of, 53, 54–55t, 55, 56t
pressure ulcers, 6, 33–34, 46–48, 61, 63–64, 86, 106–7
Preston, J., 91
private costs, 4
process efficiency, 84–85, 85f
process measures, 20, 23, 26, 47, 59–60, 61
production functions, 37–39, 39t
productive efficiency, 81, 84–85, 85f
prospective payments, 18, 59, 62, 81–82
psychiatric disorders, 13–14, 42–44
psychoactive medications, 34–36

Quality Assessment Index (Gustafson), 19–20
quality assurance, 21, 51–52, 55, 57
quality efficiency, 87t, 87–89, 88f, 108, 110
quality of care, 6–11, 10t, 105
quality of care measurement model, 85–86, 86f

race, 12–14, 13t, 105
Ramsay, J., 25, 28
Rantz, M., 60
Rantz measurement model, 24
regional location: as quality of care variable, 6, 105; in resident outcome study, 62–64, 67, 68t, 72–73t, 75, 107; telemedicine and, 91. *See also* size, metropolitan
registered nurses (RNs), 7, 36, 76–80, 83
regulations, state, 17–18, 31–32, 78
rehabilitative care, 59–60, 63–64, 67–73, 68t, 70f, 71f, 72–73t, 74–75
Reinsch, N. L., 91
resident assessment: pressure ulcer examination and, 47–48, 51, 53, 54–55t, 56t, 57, 107; staffing and, 9, 12, 61, 79
Resident Assessment Protocols (RAPs), 47
resident case mix, 21
resident-centered care, 43, 110
resident characteristics, 27
resident integrity, 39–41, 106
resident outcomes, 86; components of, 28, 29–30t
resident outcome study: conclusions of, 73–75, 107; methodology of, 63–67; overview of, 59–60; research related to, 61–63; results of, 67–73, 68t, 70f, 71f, 72–73t
resident satisfaction, 6
Residents' Bill of Rights, 77–78
resource dependence theory, 109
respite programs, 44
restraint devices: in pressure ulcer examination, 52, 54–55t, 56t, 58; and quality of care, 33–34, 79, 113; and quality of care measurement model, 86; in resident outcome study, 61–64, 107
Rhodes, E., 84
Rosen, E., 90
rural nursing homes, 14–16, 44–45, 106

Sainfort, F., 24, 28
Salancik, G., 109

satisfaction, resident, 6
Seblega, B. K., 76
Selznick, P., 109
simulation and optimization, 96, 97f, 99–100, 100–101, 108
size, metropolitan: in expanded structure-process-outcome model, 28; as quality of care variable, 6, 14–16, 105, 106; in resident outcome study, 62–63, 67, 68t, 72–73t, 74; telemedicine and, 92. *See also* rural nursing homes
Sloane, P. D., 17, 42-43
speech therapy, 43
staff: communication skills of, 11–12, 42, 105, 110–11; and hours per resident day, 7, 17, 42, 51, 53, 61; minimal levels of, 37-39, 76-80, 95, 107; optimal levels of, 79; training for, 12, 94-96. *See also* nurse staffing; staff mix
staff mix: deficiency citations and, 36, 76–77, 106; efficiency and, 81–83; in expanded structure-process-outcome model, 28; facility size and, 41; medication errors and, 35; and minimum staff levels, 76–80; prospective payments and, 18; quality efficiency and, 85–86; as quality factor, 7, 11; resident outcomes and, 59–60; rural nursing homes and, 14–15, 44. *See also* nurse staffing
state-level measurement models, 17–18, 31–32
state regulations, 17–18, 31–32, 78
statistical analysis: informatics research and, 96, 97f, 98–99, 108; pressure ulcer examination and, 51–53; and resident outcome study, 65–71, 73–75; and technical efficiency study, 84–88
Stevenson, D. G., 7
Stevenson, J., 25
stroke, 43
structure measurements, 21, 23, 26, 60
structure-process-outcome measurement models: Donabedian and others, 23–25; expanded (Unruh/Wan), 23f, 23, 27–31, 57, 60, 73; expansion of, 25–27; as framework, 106, 108–9
Swan, J. H., 41, 109
system membership. *See* chain affiliation

task technology fit theory, 94f, 94
Teaching Nursing Home program, 95–96, 101–3
technical efficiency, 81, 87t, 87–89, 88f, 101f, 108, 110
technology acceptance model (TAM), 93f, 93
Teeri, S., 40–41
telemedicine, 90–95, 108
Thomas, R. J., 91–92
total economic efficiency, 81, 84–85, 85f
training, staff, 12, 94–96
translational research, 96, 97f, 100, 108
Turner, J. W., 91–92
two-level measurement models, 18, 31–32

Unruh, L. Y.: 2004, 9, 23, 25, 28, 30, 60; 2006, 18, 34, 62, 86; 2008, 4, 82, 83
Unruh and Wan structure-process-outcome model, 23f, 23, 27–31, 57, 60, 73
urinary tract infections, 86
U.S. Bureau of Health Professions, 50
U.S. Department of Health and Human Services, 2, 7, 20, 46, 98

visitation of residents, 41

Wan, T. T. H.: 2003, 19; 2004, 9, 23, 25, 28, 30, 60; 2005, 10, 31; 2006, 18, 34, 62, 86, 96; 2007, 4, 109; 2008, 4, 82, 83
Wang, C., 2
WebMD.com, 90, 92, 104, 108. *See also* ehealth
Wogen, S. E., 83, 84
Wright, D., 91

X-efficiency, 81–82

Zhang, N. J.: 2004, 37; 2005, 10, 31; 2006, 18, 34, 37–39, 62, 86, 95; 2007, 4, 109; 2008, 2, 4, 10, 82, 83, 91–95
Zimmerman's Quality Assessment Index, 20

About the Authors

Thomas T. H. Wan, Ph.D., M.H.S. is director of the Doctoral Program in Public Affairs and professor of public affairs, health management and informatics at the College of Health and Public Affairs and is professor of medical education at the College of Medicine, University of Central Florida (UCF). He serves as an associate dean for research at the College of Health and Public Affairs, UCF. Professor Wan received a B.A. in sociology from Tunghai University, Taiwan; an M.A. and a Ph.D. in sociology and demography from the University of Georgia; and a M.H.S. from the Johns Hopkins University School of Public Health, where he was also an NIH postdoctoral fellow. His more than 30 years in academia encompass faculty positions at Cornell University, the University of Maryland Baltimore County, and Virginia Commonwealth University. His research interests include healthcare informatics research, outcomes evaluation, gerontological health, and long-term care research.

Gerald-Mark Breen, M.A., Ph.D. (posthumous), was a research associate in the Doctoral Program in Public Affairs of the College of Health and Public Affairs at the University of Central Florida. He earned his M.A. in communication from the University of Oklahoma and had undergraduate degrees in psychology and criminal justice from the University of Alaska–Fairbanks. He completed his doctoral studies at UCF. His research spanned a spectrum of health services including doctor-patient communication, telemedicine and ehealth services, and patient-centric care practices. He also conducted secondary research in emergency management and government/political protection, as well as journalism studies as they relate to ethical standards.

Ning Jackie Zhang, M.D., Ph.D., M.P.H., is an associate professor in the Doctoral Program of Public Affairs and the Department of Health Management and Informatics of the College of Health and Public Affairs, at the University of Central Florida (UCF). He is also the graduate coordinator of the program and director of the Health Informatics Lab at UCF. He obtained his doctoral degree from the Department of Health Administration, Medical College of Virginia at Virginia Commonwealth University. His research interests are in clinical outcomes research, long-term care research, emergency medical services, and health informatics.

Lynn Unruh, Ph.D., R.N., is an associate professor in the Department of Health Management and Informatics at the University of Central Florida. Professor Unruh received a B.S. in nursing from the University of Illinois and a Ph.D. in economics from the University of Notre Dame. She is also a licensed health care risk manager in the state of Florida. Her research is in the following areas: nurse staffing in hospitals and nursing homes; the relationship between nurse staffing and quality, patient safety, and costs of patient care; the nursing workforce (measuring, assessing supply and demand, forecasting); the work environment in hospitals and nursing homes; and the responses of hospitals and nursing homes to reimbursement, regulatory, and market forces. She has received funding from the Agency for Healthcare Research and Quality, the Florida Center for Nursing, the National Institute of Nursing Research, the National Science Foundation, and the Robert Wood Johnson Foundation.